DEFEAT IT!

*A Woman's Guide To Crushing Life's Challenges
And Finally Living The Fit Life*

Free Transformation Workbook Included

By Dali Burgado, CPT
CEO, DEFEAT IT, LLC
Dali Burgado Fitness
Certified Personal Trainer, NCCPT
Certified Weight Management Specialist, NCCPT
Certified Group Fitness Instructor, NCCPT

A Woman's Motivational Guidebook and Workbook.

Copyright © 2017 by Dali Burgado

Copyright Notice

Copyright © 2017 Dali Burgado

Editing by Monique Kendrick, Red Ink'd, LLC and Dali Burgado, Defeat It, LLC
Cover Photography by Luis Burgado, Think Big International, LLC
Cover Design by Luis Burgado, Think Big International, LLC
Interior Design by Dali Burgado, Defeat It, LLC

Table of Contents

By Dali Burgado, CPT

Acknowledgements and Dedication

There are so many people I'd love to thank for inspiring me to get this book done. First, I'd like to thank my daughter, Christine, for being the first one in the immediate family to have authored, illustrated *and* published a book, "The Princess and the Dragon," at the sweet age of 6 in September 2011. At the time, she was Virginia's youngest author. And this wouldn't have been possible without my husband's skills and encouragement. He is the creativity behind my analytical brain. Thank you, Luis Burgado, for the amazing book cover, and thank you for believing in me even when I doubted myself!

I'd also like to thank several of my mentors — funny enough that three of my mentors are all named AJ! Thank you, AJ Mihrazd, for all the motivation, dedication, and being a great example to follow. Thank you, AJ Rivera, for being an amazing role model and for the trainings. You both inspire me daily. AJ Silver, thank you for the spiritual direction, advice, and keeping my eyes fixed on Jesus. Thank you to coaches Pat Pilla and Celeste Rains-Turk for the pep talks and advice when I needed it! They were always on time! I'm also so grateful for all the support and friends made in my certification journey with the National Council for Certified Personal Trainers (NCCPT), including Kevin D. Starkey!

To my editor, Monique Kendrick. I'm so grateful to have met you. Thank you for the great and thorough review of the first drafts of *Defeat It!* I'm looking forward to working on many more books with you! Thank you, ShaRhonda Brown for LimeLight for the beautifully done make-up for this book cover!

And thank you Father in Heaven for choosing me to be a light and giving me the courage to inspire every single day.

I dedicate this book to every woman struggling to defeat self-doubt, past failures, and let go of past baggage. You are unique, valuable, and like no one else. You're here for a special reason, and I hope that these words will breathe renewed hope, energy, and motivation to help you slay whatever you need to defeat! This is for you!

Download your free Defeat It! workbook as well as all the online resources mentioned in the book here:

https://defeatitbook.com/workbook

Remember to join the "Defeat It! Book" Community on Facebook!

https://www.facebook.com/defeatitbook

Introduction

I'm so excited about this book. It's always been a dream of mine to make my mark on the world by authoring a book that will help women feel better about themselves in every aspect of life. Over time, I've grown to be the woman, leader, and person of strong faith that I am today; however, it took a lot and many challenges and temporary defeats to shape who I am emotionally, spiritually, and physically.

Defeat It! is more than just a fitness book. It encourages you into deep reflection, engages you to think about your goals, where you want to be, and what needs to change for you to defeat what holds you back from being your healthiest.

Defeat It! is also the story of several strong women, including myself, and how we shaped our stories or journeys to *defeat* whatever obstacles came our way. We are telling the stories of the moments that helped us begin our physical transformations, the challenges we overcame and how we overcame them, as well as life changing lessons learned. My goal with the second half of the book is to share stories of victory with you so that you can defeat whatever is holding you back from loving yourself more and becoming the best version of you yet.

By Dali Burgado, CPT

The first 9 chapters of this book include both my life and fitness experiences, lessons learned, and advice on how you can either begin your fitness journey or continue to build momentum towards your current journey and best self! The first few chapters contain written exercises to help you reflect and find your deep desire to live your fullest, healthiest life. It also includes motivation strategies and tips. I encourage you to write as you think and avoid censoring yourself. Write freely.

Whether you struggle with food, mindset, exercise, or spirituality, *Defeat It!* will help inspire you to think about your current situation and provide different strategies to help you defeat *your* "it"!

Here's to victory and positive life-change!

I'd love to hear stories of how this book

has helped you in your fitness journey and

be able to share your story on my website.

Please reach out to me at

daliburgadofitness@daliburgado.com to

share your victories with me!

Chapter 1: From Defeated to Defeat It!

*"From victory we learn little, from defeat -
everything."*
— Jeffrey Fry, Former Baseball Player

The hardest part of any journey is getting started. And it's easy for most people to feel defeated before they even begin. However, it's from temporary defeat that we learn the most about ourselves and our true capabilities. Read the following social media status update that caught my eye.

Every time I watch her videos I am amazed and think, 'Okay, I've got to go back. Take that first step...(again). It's the journey that counts.' But it sure would be amazing to progress...a lot! (Truth be told, I also think I should just throw in the towel!)

\- Facebook Friends' Status Update

"Well - saw this as I'm about to go do my exercise for the week ... feeling a lot inadequate now ... mine looks nothing like that."

\- Response to that update

I'm amazed by this emotion in the status update from a friend. She was talking about a video she watched with some very advanced yoga moves and how it inspired her, but at the same time it defeated her. To her, it wasn't where she needed to start, and she couldn't see herself doing those advanced moves. She understood that it takes many little steps to get there, but she almost instantly felt defeated. This led me to think more about this topic and even the focus of this book.

> Comparison is the thief of joy! You
>
> shouldn't compare your fitness journey to
>
> anyone else's!

As we look at the example set by my friend's social media post, not only was she defeated, but she was unknowingly comparing her current fitness level to an advanced yoga teacher's fitness level. By doing this, she is missing the fact that this teacher very likely took a while to become who she is today. She's feeling she'll never measure up because after all, there is some hope that success should be instant. Subconsciously, she believes that fast progress should be possible and that might motivate her to begin.

Always remember this. Comparison is the thief of joy! You shouldn't compare your fitness journey to anyone else's! You have unique experiences, talents, strengths, and weaknesses. There is only one you. You may not be able to perform advanced yoga moves, swan dive and touch your toes, lift two 25 lb. dumbbells and lunge, or do burpees right now, but over time you will build your strength, stamina, and self-confidence. Yes, it takes *time*! Don't get side-tracked by the false claims of instant progress. The media and false marketing are to blame for this big ole lie! Progress is just what it is, incremental!

...when you end up comparing your day 1

to someone else's day 1,000, you start

seeing reasons why you will never measure

up and feel like you want to quit before

you begin. But when you compare yourself

to who you were yesterday that's where

the real magic happens!

Not only that, when you end up comparing your day 1 to someone else's day 1,000, you start seeing reasons why you will never measure up and feel like you want to quit before you begin. But when you compare yourself to who you were yesterday that's where the real magic happens! You start to see the small possibilities and focus on small improvements.

Remember this. You're only in competition with yourself. Keep that in mind as you begin your fitness journey, whether you're starting out or simply looking for something new to do to take you to that next step in your journey towards your goal.

Remember this. You're only in competition

with yourself. Keep that in mind as you

begin your fitness journey, whether you're

starting out or simply looking for

something new to do to take you to that

next step in your journey towards your

goal.

Instead of feeling like my friend, would you rather *Defeat It!?* What does defeating *it* mean for you? It could mean defeating the negative self-talk, defeating unhealthy eating patterns, defeating the lack of motivation to make a change, defeating the anxiety with going to the gym, or defeating putting yourself second instead of first.

By Dali Burgado, CPT

Write down a few things you've been struggling with lately when it comes to your health and fitness and *put a star by the strongest one*. That one is your "it."

_____

_____

_____

_____

_____

_____

Whatever *it* is you're trying to defeat my goal is to help you squash that one thing that is keeping you from living your healthiest life! Let's get started!

The hardest thing is starting any fitness routine without feeling like you need to throw in the towel. Once you begin, it gets so much easier. The little steps add up over time, and before you know it, you've formed a habit. But what's going to sustain you? What's going to keep you going?

You need a turning point in your life, something to spark the flame, something to help you start afresh or begin in the first place. Instead of thinking about some huge insurmountable goal, think about small goals and small steps that'll take you in the right direction because fitness is a journey, and every one of us has our own unique journey.

And you know what? You get to write that journey. Yes! Every decision you make will paint the story. Every decision every day adds up over time creating a new and healthier you. You are the author of your lifestyle!

As you continue reading, I hope you learn from my experiences and the experiences of other women who were interviewed for this book and take that turning point that will lead you on the path to your healthiest and best self!

You are the author of your lifestyle!

I still struggle with communicating my feelings verbally and expressing my emotions. In the chapters that follow, I'm going to do my best to describe all the events that shaped who I am now and how you can take these experiences to shape who you want to become. Welcome to the journey to *Defeat It!*

By Dali Burgado, CPT

Finding Your Turning Point

"Remember no man is really defeated unless he is discouraged."

— *Bruce Lee, American martial artist, actor, philosopher, filmmaker*

Each of us have turning points, or what I like to call "defining moments", that shape who we become and what we prioritize in life. Read on to learn what mine was and start thinking about your defining moments or turning points. In the final chapters of this book, you'll see the defining moments of four other women as well.

The Turning Point That Sparked My Flame

It was a warm late summer morning, on Friday, August 31st, 2012. I was on my way to work, and as usual took the back roads from my home. It was a gorgeous day. Since my Civic was in the shop, I had to drive the big Expedition that morning.

I was nearly five minutes away from work when I approached a windy road, my vehicle dipped into gravel, and my car lost traction. Suddenly, I couldn't even manage to keep the vehicle going straight after efforts to steer my way back to safety. The vehicle started to swerve like it had a life of its own. Doing a complete flip, my hunky Expedition landed in a grassy field, luckily right side up.

As my vehicle flipped, my life flashed before my eyes. My kids, husband, I thought *'my story couldn't be over'.* I said a quick flash prayer, "God be with me."

I felt as if I was protected in a bubble. I know I flipped over at least once. But I heard bystanders tell the troopers that I had flipped over twice. Either way, I thank God that I landed safely in that grassy area and that I didn't hit anything or anyone.

The left side of my vehicle - driver's side - was totaled. And the only thing saving me besides God's angels was a piece of sod embedded in the top left-hand corner of the windshield. Had that glass broken, I would have been dead.

That morning, I was the most grateful woman alive. I got a second chance at life! It made me realize all the unhealthy patterns that I was living in my life and all the things about me that I wasn't proud of. My near-death experience made me take a close look at myself and the habits I needed to change. I had plenty of unhealthy habits in my relationship, as well as within myself and my lack of exercising and eating. These habits needed to change if I wanted to show God my appreciation for another chance at life and living to my fullest potential.

That morning, the brave fire and rescue volunteers carefully took me out of the vehicle and an ambulance rushed me to the nearest hospital. I was in and out with no injuries- except for a little bruise on my left thigh. I was pretty much untouched. My vehicle was totaled, but my life wasn't. Praise God my Civic wasn't on the road that day and I was alive and well.

I didn't realize it that day, but that day I defeated living a mediocre life and chose to live my life to my greatest potential.

What's YOUR Turning Point?

Unfortunately, for many of us, including myself, it takes something huge — a death in the family, a near-death experience, a divorce, or a major life-changing event — to help you change direction with your health and fitness. For me, my defining moment was that car accident at the age of 32 that beautiful August morning.

My kids were still young. I wouldn't say I was fit, but I wasn't in the worst shape ever. While I was satisfied in my skin, I was doing things in my life that were unhealthy, causing myself unnecessary stress, and I was not active. I needed a stress outlet and had no one I could talk to. I was not eating as healthy as I used to. I hadn't exercised in years. And more importantly, my husband and I were having martial issues that needed to be resolved. I was a ticking time bomb. Can you relate to a crazy time in your life?

Take these turning point stories in your life and make them your defining moments. These moments will change your course, and you can use them as fuel! Don't wait for something catastrophic to change your life. After my accident, I wanted to just go all-out with my fitness because I was grateful for a new chance! I also wanted to be around for my kids for as long as possible. My family at that point became my motivation to want to be super healthy so that I could be around for them as long as God allowed me to. God saved me from that accident, and I was not going to let my second chance go to waste!

The Monday after the accident, I brought my gym clothes to work and began walking on the treadmill at the work gym during my lunch hour. From then, I walked and jogged and then started running outside with a friend. Before I knew it, I registered to run my first 5K (3.2 miles) the following spring and then began training for my first 10-mile race that summer. I never was a runner, so it was a challenge. It was the first time I had trained for anything. While I finished near the end on that 10-mile race, I was so grateful that I could complete it!

I spent the next two years training one day a week with a personal trainer and following a series of workout plans. When that trainer moved, I began creating my own training plans and continued to soak up all the fitness knowledge I could. Other ladies in the gym began asking me what I was doing to build lean muscle. As others noticed my physical transformation, I was getting leaner and stronger, even the "fit crowd" in the gym was asking me questions. People were following my workouts, and I knew I had to get certified and help other women get fit. As a result, in July of 2015, I became a Certified Personal Trainer through the National Council for Certified Personal Trainers (NCCPT).

As I reflected on my story, I realize it was that one car accident and God sparing my life that made me go into the direction of Personal Training and away from the Information Technology direction I'd been going. I wanted to encourage and inspire women to get fit. This was *my* true defining moment. And defining moments don't need to be near catastrophic!

Another defining moment for me was my experience with my third pregnancy at age 36, when I gained a significant amount of weight quickly, which I'll share more about soon.

What will be your defining moment? Will it be you gaining 20 pounds in a month? Will it be the depression you've been feeling because your clothes don't fit the way they used to? Will it be your crying in the closet looking at the clothes that no longer fit? Will it be a recent break-up or a divorce, a new job, a vacation that you're planning in six months, a wedding or a reunion?

There are so many defining moments in our lives that can change our habits and that can help light a fire in you to form new and healthier habits.

What's your defining moment?

What events and feelings have recently transpired that you can use to fuel your motivation to get fit? **Write down your defining moment (or moments).**

_____

_____

_____

_____

_____

_____

_____

Now, I encourage you to think about your true motivation to get healthy. **_Why now?_** What's going to motivate you to begin? Write your thoughts below. What's the emotional or financial cost to you and your loved ones if you don't begin now?

_____

_____

_____

_____

_____

_____

_____

We'll touch on more things to help you get motivated later. But right now, look at your life and where you want to be and start writing down a few things that you can do now to help you prioritize yourself and your health first. It can be having more "me time," eating healthier meals, adding more exercise into your daily plans, talking to family more often, planning a family vacation, etc. Schedule these into your calendar and set a reminder to get them done!

I will prioritize my health by doing these things this week:

1) _____

2) _____

3) _____

Chapter 2: Your Relationship with You

"Whatever you do
be gentle with yourself.
You don't just live
in this world
or your home
or your skin. You also live
in someone's eyes."
— Sanober Khan, Mumbai-based poet and
freelance writer

The strongest relationship to work on is the one you have with you! I love the quote above because it gets to the heart that others depend on us, and we can be role models to others, especially those closest to us, like our children, for example.

However, as women we tend to either put ourselves first, selfishly, or we put others first to our demise. Whether it's, our husband, kids, or even careers, we prioritize other things and people before we even think about ourselves. And this doesn't leave us with "me time" or workout time! Sometimes we don't feel worthy of putting ourselves first. And sometimes we hold onto past baggage that drag us down and enables us to put everyone else first. All the while we are distracted from really working on ourselves. Realize this if this sounds like you. Be kind to yourself. Work on you.

We don't realize that by working on the relationship with *ourselves*, we become a better and less grouchy wife, a better friend, more loving mom, and a more competent career woman. So, not only do our relationships with others get better, but the relationship with ourselves gets better.

Let me tell you how it was for me and my evolution. For as long as I can remember, I've been very focused, driven, and ready to tackle challenges. And this did not change after marriage or children. But this drive came at a cost. I was selfish. I was all about me in a completely unhealthy way.

During college, I put on more than the freshman 15 times two. After college graduation, I managed to lose about 10 pounds living on my own, making healthier decisions, cooking better and avoiding all the bad food that I used to eat as a kid growing up with my family. I thought about myself often. In my mid-twenties, I met someone very special. And he became my husband.

When I first got married and had my first two children, I don't think I was ready *emotionally*. I was very self-centered, as most of us unknowingly are, and I put my feelings and myself first. I got married at the age of 25 and was 26 by the time I had my second child. I was so determined to make my home business thrive even while caring for two children under the age of two. All that pressure on myself stressed me out.

I worked long hours, sacrificed family time, and avoided date nights with the husband. I was a slave to my work, and I saw nothing wrong with chasing "success." My relationships suffered because of that. Subconsciously and emotionally, I don't think I was ready to have kids and be the wife my husband needed. My desire to work, work, work and chase success really took precedence over my health and my family in my mid 20's and beyond. I frequently ate at gas stations and fast food restaurants, and I did not workout. So, it wasn't the best of times for me and my health or my marriage.

In my 30's, I changed completely. And I owe it to that car accident that forever changed me. It pushed me to see who I was as a wife and mom. For you, some other stressful event or temporary defeat may trigger you to self-reflect and see how you can love yourself, your family, and others more. It's during those moments in the deep valleys where we grow most.

It's during those moments in the deep

valleys where we grow most.

I learned from my mistakes and how my family suffered from my obsession with chasing success and wanting to be so successful. So instead of prioritizing money and work, I became passionate about my health and fitness, and that helped me reduce stress at work and at home. It made me a more proactive woman. That passion later evolved into a newfound passion for helping others regain control of their health and lives as well as a passion for God and family.

Today, I'm prioritizing that very passion for helping others through life-change with my fitness business, through breakthroughs with my coaching, and by authoring personal transformational books.

> It's okay to not have it all together. It's
>
> okay to want to look and feel better. It's
>
> okay to prioritize you first because you
>
> can't serve at your best when you're not
>
> healthy. When you prioritize your health,
>
> you're prioritizing yourself as a mom,
>
> business or career woman, and wife.

So, work on the relationship with you. Recognize when you're not giving your family and spouse the attention needed to thrive in relationship.

And you know what? It's okay to not have it "all together." It's okay to want to look and feel better. It's okay to prioritize *you* first because you can't serve at your best when you're not healthy. When you prioritize your health, you're prioritizing yourself as a mom, business or career woman, and wife. Your ability to take care of your children, family, and work or business will increase. Your happiness will also increase exponentially due to the added energy.

So, what can you do to prioritize your health right now – and not only your physical health but your emotional and mental health? These are things that women struggle with at any age. Think about each of the following areas and what you can do to prioritize your health in the upcoming weeks.

I will do these things for each of these categories:

My Emotional Health

Who can you contact when you're in a slump?

1) _____

2) _____

What can you do to feel better now?

1) _____

2) _____

Add these in your calendar! Set a reminder to get them done.

My Physical Health

What can I do to move more throughout your day? What small steps can I take today and tomorrow to start or get better with my current fitness level?

1) _____

2) _____

3) _____

Add these in your calendar! Set a reminder to get them done.

<u>My Mental Health</u>

It's okay to cry, talk to someone, and feel angry or upset. What can you let go of this week? What can you do to feel better?

1) _____

2) _____

Add these in your calendar! Set a reminder to get them done.

You are worthy of greater things, and you

deserve time to de-stress!

Be Completely Honest with Yourself

One thing that will help you especially with your mental and emotional health is being completely honest with yourself and how happy you are with your current decisions and where your life is headed. One thing that can wreak havoc on our minds is forcing ourselves to believe something that's untrue like the feeling that you may be unworthy of better things or that you don't deserve time to yourself. You are worthy of greater things, and you deserve time to de-stress! After all, this important "me time" helps keep you sane!

And if we're talking honesty, ask yourself these questions. Are you truly happy in your current body? Are the decisions you're currently making daily moving you closer to or further away from your goals? Do you love who you see in the mirror? Do you love more than just the physical – I mean, the soul staring back at you?

I recently had to be real with myself. All I had to do was look at pictures and listen to my doctor. I hit my heaviest weight during my last pregnancy. At age 36, I became pregnant once again, 10 years after what I thought would have been my last pregnancy. I became depressed. I hit one of my lowest emotional moments in that first month or two of pregnancy and as a result, I resorted to emotional eating. Like so many of us, pregnant or not, when we get depressed we suppress our feelings with comfort in food.

Within the first 4 weeks after learning I was pregnant, I gained 13 lbs. I knew I had to stop gaining weight so quickly, but hey, I was pregnant. That's what a pregnant woman is supposed to do – eat for two!

No, not really.

I was given doctor's orders to monitor my weight gain because it was too much in a month for my small pregnant frame; I'm 4'11". I absolutely knew I was heading in the wrong direction at that point. I got real with myself!

By Dali Burgado, CPT

Before becoming pregnant in 2016, I had gotten to the point where I had the most muscle. I had been working out consistently since 2012. I worked hard throughout my four-year fitness journey. I became trim, and I felt sexy and the healthiest I'd ever been, but after the pregnancy, I took things 180 degrees. I stopped eating healthy, and I stopped going to the gym. *I felt defeated.*

Food became my go-to once the depression kicked in. Why was I so depressed? What was wrong with me? Well, I was approaching my late 30s, my husband and I didn't plan the pregnancy, and I feared what was to come. I feared that at the healthiest in my life, I would lose my fit body for good. Yup. I would never get my body back! I was discouraged. I was sitting in my pity party. *I didn't know it then, but I had to defeat my fear and the negative self-talk in my head!*

You see, I started thinking so negatively that now my emotions and mindset were in the dumps. I started eating chips, chocolate ice cream, and chocolate chip cookies every night. I began packing on the pounds. And none were from the pregnancy.

When my doctor said I needed to slow my roll and control my weight gain, it became yet another defining moment for me! At that moment, I thought to myself, *'What's wrong with me? I'm supposed to be a personal trainer. Why am I not doing what I need to do?'*

I didn't like it. I didn't like the way I was feeling, and I knew that if I didn't take control of my pregnancy and what I ate, I *definitely* wouldn't get my body back. And there was no way I was going to be the unfit personal trainer! I had to practice what I preached! I had to reconcile my beliefs and get it right again! So, I decided to follow my own advice and I began working out again. I had stopped working out for about eight weeks, and it was within that short amount of time that I started really looking unhealthy and feeling heavy. That just fueled a spark in me to start taking control of my life again.

The doctor's orders motivated me to get back to working out and eating healthier. I dropped the daily chips and ice cream. I snacked on healthier options and kept my portions under control. The portion control also helped me avoid that pesky pregnancy heartburn! From about month 4 (second trimester onwards), I went back to working out three times per week (less than I was used to) and began controlling the weight gain. My goal was to gain under 25 lbs. total for my small frame. I gained 21 overall, and by the third trimester, during my last 4 doctor visits I maintained the same body weight even though the baby kept growing!

What if I had not gotten the courage to defeat my fear?

After the baby was born, I followed a clean, high-fiber diet, and I began to see the post-pregnancy pounds melt away. I began working out post-pregnancy at week 4. By the end of post-pregnancy week 8, I lost 29 lbs., and by week 12

I lost 33. Total to date, I've lost 40 lbs. post-baby, and I'm the trimmest I've been since my teenage years and still strong. Of course, I'm not perfect, and I still have stretch marks, but I love my new post-mom body, and I feel just as sexy as before.

When you're pregnant, so many people tell you that you're eating for two and encourage you to eat and eat. And that's bull. If you speak to your doctor, he or she will tell you that all you need is an extra 300-500 calories or so during pregnancy and that is mainly in trimesters two and three (Farmer, Randall and Aziz 2014), which amounts to an extra snack or two or a small meal. So, you are not eating for two, you are eating for yourself and a growing fetus who will become a baby.

If you're pregnant, use your pregnancy as an opportunity for you to eat healthier. Not only for you, but for your baby too! People will tell you, "Oh, it's all right, go and eat all you want. You're eating for two anyway!" but don't listen to them.

So be completely honest with yourself. How satisfied are you with the way you look in pictures now and in the mirror? Why? Do you look in the mirror and something in you just wants to cringe? If so, that's your deepest self-telling you that you need to start doing things to change. Don't wait for doctor's orders! Use your defining moments as fuel to become your best self!

Reflection Time

What moments of honesty came to mind as you read this chapter? What things can you begin doing to improve your relationship with you this week?

_____

_____

_____

_____

_____

_____

_____

_____

_____

_____

_____

_____

Chapter 3: Focus on the Journey and Plan

*"We may run, walk, stumble, drive, or fly, but let
us never lose sight of the reason for the journey,
or miss a chance to see a rainbow on the way."*

— Gloria Gaither, Christian Songwriter

Put One Foot In Front Of The Other

Fitness and life are journeys. Success is never instant. And it's beautiful and encouraging to see the small milestones along the way. It's the journey that makes us. But most of us want results now like my friend in the beginning of this book. We live in the culture of *now*.

It's the journey that makes us.

Commercials and ads attempt to convince you that you need the latest health and beauty products now and that these programs will provide maximum results (and I'd dare to say most don't). This is also true in the fitness industry with fad diets to the next silly gadget that won't get you any closer to your fitness or weight loss goal. So many of us spend our money on the "now".

But the "now" has a lot more to do with our emotional, physical and psychological factors and not the promise of that very product. Often, when we decide that we need something, and we chose to spend our hard-earned cash on it, it's because we associate more pain with our current situation and see the product as a solution to alleviate that pain. The product is viewed as a false sense of hope to make us feel better about ourselves and regain some control of our situation. We rationalize and convince ourselves that we need the product, but we also fool ourselves into thinking that progress should be fast, especially when we spend a lot of money on a product or service.

> Your fitness journey is all a process, and in
>
> that process, there will be progress!

That's when things get iffy. You see, there is change that needs to take place *internally*, whether it's dropping past baggage, believing in ourselves, learning more about life or health, or applying ourselves and really deciding that enough is enough and making a 100% commitment to get stuff done! We first need to go through an internal transformation before we get to the outward transformation! This is where you start to take arms and defeat what's holding you back!

What's more is that your fitness journey is all a process, and in that process, there will be progress! But how do we learn to accept that we should look for progress instead of the instant results and gratification promised by so many marketed products? We shift our focus! We think *longer-term!*

I know, it doesn't sound sexy, right? But when you're focused on the next fitness and nutrition goal and milestones, you're well on your way to living your fittest life.

> We first need to go through an internal
>
> transformation before we get to the
>
> outward transformation!

It's tough for us to think ahead and consider goal-setting in any area of life, and this holds true for fitness. But start to think about your life three months in advance. Think about your life six months from now and within the next year. How will your life change after weeks of adding better choices into your life?

Start thinking like a high school senior again. Back when you were in high school, you had to set deadlines, plan, talk to your guidance counselor, and pay your dues in order to be ready for graduation. Think of your goal as that graduation. What needs to be done for you to get there? You need to plan *now* for where you want to be three months from now and beyond.

Even if we just look at planning everything we need to do that day at work and at home. Without a plan for the day, or a checklist of some sort, it's so easy for us to let our day run us instead of us running our day! Well, think about living like that every day over three months. That's how most Americans live when it comes to most goals, including fitness, day-by-day.

> Without a plan for the day, or a checklist of
>
> some sort, it's so easy for us to let our day
>
> run us instead of us running our day!

We think, "Well, if I get the workout in today, I'll get it in. No big deal" or "I'll eat all I want and get back to my diet next week," without considering how this continued pattern will look like 3-6 months down the future if left unchecked. Progress starts with a plan. One day at a time. One week at a time. Positive decision making over weeks, months, and beyond will yield positive results.

Think of it this way – if you start a new gym membership yet don't have a plan in place, what happens? You end up doing the treadmill for two weeks and quit. The reason is you had no plan on how to get from point A to point B. Unless, you were truly helped by gym staff and were offered and invested in a personal training plan, you wouldn't know what to do other than cardio. However, if you had a roadmap and followed it over the course of 12 weeks (3 months), chances are you'd see the results you were hoping for, even if not exact. This is the power of a plan!

So, start planning for the long game or the long-term. Whether this means a month from now or three months, six months, or longer, you should begin thinking about your long-term health, life, and personal and family goals.

Progress starts with a plan. One day at a

time. One week at a time. Positive decision

making over weeks, months, and beyond

will yield positive results.

One of the crazy examples on how we don't think long-term, especially with food, is a post that a friend posted on Facebook. She posts:

"Why do I do it to myself? I see something and say, that looks good, but it's going to hurt my stomach. I eat it anyway, saying the whole time, this is so good, but I'm going to be so sick. And of course, when the gut-wrenching pain comes, I say, what was I thinking? Feeling disgusted...

My response to that was, try this:

Focus on the pain afterwards instead of the temporary pleasure. Think long-term health. You get better by multiplying one small decision over and over every day. Drink tons of water. If you're craving junk, you're likely

dehydrated.

So, you see in this example with the subject of food, we want that instant gratification, whether it's satisfying that sweet tooth or that savory tooth or whatever. Instead of thinking about how that one decision made now may impact us later, whether that's the next few hours or the next week or month or months to come, we want instant satisfaction.

Start thinking about what it is that you're eating now. *Begin to journal your food choices.* Add that up week over week over week. If you can see that one food decision leading you to worse health later down the road, then start cutting back one thing at a time. You can cut back on one thing a week. Or if you want to reach a certain goal, cut back two things a week of whatever junk food you're eating.

There is power in thinking long-term. Even if it's a small decision now, adding these "small" decisions make big impact. Start thinking about how those little decisions over time add up and will impact your health.

If you're thinking, *'Dali. But I struggle with food cravings'*, there will be more later about how you can cope with that!

"Finding the Time"

I get this question often. *'Dali, how do I find time to work out?'* Or, *'how do you find time to work out?'*

First, you must make your health a priority. Make exercise and eating well a priority. When you make something a priority, you will make the time for it in your schedule.

Once you complete your *Defeat It! Workbook,* you'll be fired up about planning and finding time to get fit!

Are you a morning person or not? Fit in at least 25 minutes of non-negotiable "me time" to workout. And plan your meals in advance.

Begin now by blocking out 25 minutes in your calendar at least 3x a week where you will commit to "me time." You can take a walk, do yoga, stretch, jog, or workout. Just start somewhere and start moving. It can be small for now, but the harder you can push yourself to make those changes now, the easier it will be in the long term.

What three days and times will you set aside for *me time*? Do this now! And put it on your calendar of choice!

I will work out on the following days:

1) _____

2) _____

3) _____

Now, tell your significant other and closest friends and family so they know when you have your *me-time* and when not to call you!

Monday, Wednesday and Friday are good easy days to start. You only need to exercise a minimum of 3x a week, to begin seeing the benefits of an exercise program. It also gives you a recovery day in between. This is especially helpful if you're starting a new program after a long hiatus (over 6 months, for example) and if you're new to working out.

Regarding nutrition, there are several things you can do to make eating healthier easier. Purchase your groceries once a week. Plan dinner the night before or early the same day. Make a habit of defrosting your meat the night before. Delegate any prep to your kids (if they're old enough) or to your spouse.

Go to my online resources link mentioned at the beginning of the book and review my approved food and snacks list. If you're on the run and need to stop at a gas station, you may even find some healthy snacks. Have a look at my top recommendations for ideas!

Chapter 4: Being Unhealthy Doesn't Mean You Have To Be Obese

"Just because you're not sick doesn't mean you're healthy."

– Author Unknown

In my twenties, I was "chubby," but always comfortable, with my curves. I never went past a size nine. At 4'11" that's quite over, but being Puerto Rican, curvy was always the thing, and I didn't mind the curves or the extra cellulite.

It wasn't until I started working out, though, that I did feel the difference in my overall health. I felt the difference in my ability to climb up the stairs and not be winded. And I felt the difference in my body composition. I felt sexier having a looser waistline and wearing clothes that looked better on me.

So, you don't need to be obese to start getting healthier. You don't need to be heavily overweight to be unhealthy. In fact, as a young adult, I grew up with slightly overweight parents who were both diabetic and had high blood pressure. I didn't think it was normal or healthy for them to have to take pills. I knew I didn't want to take pills when I got to be their age, or at all.

My grandmother passed away from diabetes. My father has always been overweight and he too has diabetes. Both my parents and my grandparents on both sides have needed to take medicine to control hypertension, blood pressure, and diabetes. So, there is a family history of disease brought on by unhealthy eating.

As long as I lived in my mother's apartment, there were always lots of sweets in the house and plenty of fried food. Coming from a Puerto Rican household, we had Spam sandwiches, Spam omelets, or Cheese Whiz sandwiches for breakfast—all on white bread! I still reminisce about the Cheese Whiz...

...you don't need to be obese to start

getting healthier.

The healthy part of our meal was the unhealthy iceberg lettuce with a slice of tomato. Luckily, we used vinegar with a little bit of salt and pepper instead of a heavy store-bought dressing. We ate a lot of pork shoulder, fried pork chops, processed foods, sugar, soda, fast food, and food high in saturated fat and sodium. We used to eat KFC, at least once a month, but we'd eat McDonalds every Sunday after church.

We weren't very health conscious as a family of 6 at the time. It's challenging, especially when you come from a culture where all your food is either processed or fried. There's very little fiber in the standard "Newyorican" diet (New Yorkers from Puerto Rican background). And forget water. We had sugary fruit punch and orange juice to quench our thirst!

These types of food choices may not necessarily impact a woman in her early 20s. I don't think it did too much for me, but what if I continued eating that way? So being unhealthy doesn't mean you need to be obese. In my early 20's, I gained the freshman 15 and the senior 15. I carried the weight in my hips, thighs, and butt — true definition of a pear shape!

When I got out on my own, I decided that I was going to change how I cooked. I began reading labels for sodium, cholesterol, and fat content. I decided not to cook any fried foods. I began drinking water! I cut out the heavily processed foods. I cut out the excess oil. I cut out pork. I went from eating pork to eating lean meat (chicken, turkey, and fish). I wasn't much of a beef eater, but I limited red meat too.

See, you don't need to be super unsatisfied with your physical appearance to get on your health kick! If you want to avoid the medication as you age, get your energy back, reduce your stress levels, gain confidence, and feel better about yourself, you can take your defining moment(s), use them as fuel, get real with yourself, and start!

What 3 foods are you willing to let go of or severely limit this week or within the next three weeks? List them below.

I am going to give up these foods this week:

1) _____

2) _____

3) _____

Food, in my opinion, is up to 80% of the struggle when it comes to weight loss, so keep track of what you're eating. If you need a worksheet to help you get going, download my meal tracking worksheet as well as my list of top delicious whole unprocessed foods to incorporate into your diet!

And before we even think about exercise, let's take inventory of what your *views* are when it comes to food. Yes, you have some preconceived notions on what food means to you. So, let's dive into the next chapter.

Chapter 5: How Do You View Food?

"I am not a glutton - I am an explorer of food."

— *Erma Bombeck, American Humorist*

As each of us grow up, we inherit our beliefs on most things like food from our parents, guardians, and close relatives. Chances are if your parents viewed food in a certain way, you inherited those opinions. However, you can change them at any moment.

Which one are you?

Food as an Inconvenience

I have many conversations on a weekly basis with women who want to lose weight, but their "relationship" or the association they have with food is one that goes against their goals. What do I mean by this?

Several weeks ago, I asked an acquaintance how often she was eating throughout the day. The woman is a Realtor, so she's a professional who's just very, very busy. And she is so preoccupied with everything she needs to get done during the day that she skips most of her meals. She just doesn't eat enough. In conversation, she called eating "an inconvenience."

So here, we see that her association with food is negative. Since she views food as an inconvenience, she's not prioritizing feeding her body the nutrients it needs to perform at an optimal level and recover from her workouts!

In order for her to get back on track with better eating habits, she needs to change her perception of food. Instead of seeing it as an inconvenience, she needs to start seeing food as what's going to fuel her day, nourish her, and keep her healthy so that she can become a better and more productive Realtor. Having the second view of food will serve this woman better in her fitness journey. You can choose what you believe about food.

eating more often helps you stay fuller

longer so you're not overindulging and

going over your daily calories, which will

cause weight-gain.

If you can relate to this one, stop your thoughts in their tracks and have snacks handy. Set a timer if you need to. It's been debated in scientific and nutrition circles whether eating on schedule helps your metabolism. However, eating more often helps you stay fuller longer so you're not overindulging and going over your daily calories, which will cause weight-gain. And when you don't eat enough your body retains fat because fat is the best fuel source for your body when you don't have fuel (food) to keep you going. If you must, schedule food into your daily routine (or chaos)!

Comfort and Love

Do you see food as comfort? In a lot of cultures, food is a social thing. I can completely relate to this one being Hispanic and of Puerto Rican descent. Food can be a way to feel good. It's a way to celebrate being with family or being with friends. Its importance is magnified during holidays, and for Hispanic cultures it's also important even when we just have company or family over.

Be aware when you're stressed out, and

look for proactive ways to do healthier

things when you're feeling stressed such as

go for a walk, run, or head to the gym for a

workout.

In Hispanic culture, there always needs be plenty of food on the table. Food is comfort. Food is love. And we tend to share that "love" and overindulge in it with family around. Do you see food this way?

Sometimes people use that comfort and use food to feel better about themselves and about their situation. When someone is stressed as well, sometimes stress eating comes into play.

Realize when you're having these thoughts about food and start replacing these thoughts with better serving thoughts. Be aware when you're stressed out, and look for proactive ways to do healthier things when you're feeling stressed such as go for a walk, run, or head to the gym for a workout. Try meditation, talking to someone, or journaling. Avoid eating while stressed.

The Over-indulger

There are some people who see food as pure pleasure. Because food is pleasure, these individuals tend to overeat and overindulge. They will eat when they're bored and just because food tastes good and is something to do. The over-indulger uses little self-control.

Realize if this is you, and do your best to eat only until you're satisfied and not full. Most people think that you're supposed to eat until you're full, and that's not true. You're supposed to eat until your satiated. It takes time for your food to digest, and we jam pack out intestines when we overeat. If you're an over-indulger, snacking every 2.5 to 3 hours will help you here. The more frequent meals you eat throughout the day, the less hungry you will be during big meal times (i.e. lunch and dinner). And stay hydrated.

Can you think of reasons why you might over-indulge? How can you avoid over-indulging at home and at social

By Dali Burgado, CPT

gatherings? Recognize these feelings and remember you can stop yourself from going overboard.

_____

_____

_____

_____

_____

_____

The Health Nut

Then there are people who eat tree bark. I'm joking, of course. I'm referring to the health nuts. The Super Health Nut may not be getting the appropriate nutrition i.e. proteins, fiber, fats, vitamins, and minerals given food limitations. This person may view food as life, but is always on top of Dr. "So-and-So" or the latest research on what veggies or fruits are "bad for you". This person over analyzes what's good and what's bad for you. This person needs to strike a little bit of balance, and stop being so critical.

A food journal and nutritionist services can help determine if you're getting the proper nutrition in your current diet.

The Grazers

Then you have the "grass-eaters," or those who eat way too little. These are light grazers. A lot of moms fit into this category. Maybe depression gets you down, and you don't eat often. Grazers also can get too wrapped up in the daily mom activities or work grazing here and there without realizing that you skipped lunch.

Like the health nut, if you're a grazer, you're likely not getting enough essential nutrients, vitamins, and minerals. Strive to eat a breakfast and lunch even if your dinner is light. You'd also likely benefit from nutritionist services.

Fast Foodies

Then you have the fast food eaters, those who are totally unprepared and don't shop with a food list. They rely on drive-throughs for sustenance. When you're unprepared, you buy fast food often, and you eat out too much.

If you're a fast foodie, take the weekend (or any day you're off) to prepare in advance, and really look at how much money is going to fast food and eating out every month. Often, you are wasting like $300 - $500 or more. And sometimes that amounts to a whole month of grocery shopping, or it could be extra money that you could be saving or putting towards meal planning, nutrition, and personal training.

In a Nut-shell

To improve your nutritional health, you need to prepare in advance. This could mean you start shopping once a week and planning your dinners or cook several big meals you can freeze on a Sunday. I like to make big dinners twice per week that I can serve two nights in a row. You also need to recognize the association you have with food. Is it a good or bad association? Which food type do you associate yourself with most?

Begin to see food as essential fuel to make you the BEST YOU every day. Food is life. If you need to remind yourself, write a note or print this motto on your refrigerator. Food is life!

Begin to see food as essential fuel to make

you the BEST YOU every day. Food is life.

Recognize and acknowledge when you feel depressed or stressed, and stop yourself before using food as comfort when you're not hungry. If you need to, seek professional help. This habit can be a sign of uncovered or unaired emotional issues you have not dealt with and haven't let go. If you think you have a food disorder, it's best to get help now than later.

Remember, as long as you keep improving your dietary habits over time, drink enough water, and get the appropriate amount of fiber from fruits and vegetables or grains you'll stop getting cravings.

Aim for balance with your nutrition and fitness. I am not a fan of "diets". For one thing, the name has a bad and restrictive connotation, and overall has a bad rep. Most people cringe at the sound of the word and don't sustain or keep up with them. I *am* a fan of focusing on balanced nutrition and building habits over time. It's not about having a "perfect" diet but empowering yourself to know what's the healthiest option for you.

Remember, keep track of when you're thinking negatively and you when you have feelings that either make you want to eat food or make you want to skip out on food. Log your feelings in your journal if you need to, and start to plan better. Begin planning which healthy meals you're going to incorporate into your routine this week. Become a "snacker" if you're not one. If you currently snack, consider how healthy your current snacks are.

Remember, as long as you keep improving

your dietary habits over time, drink

enough water, and get the appropriate

amount of fiber from fruits and vegetables

or grains you'll stop getting cravings.

Food for thought. Can you modify a current recipe that uses red meat for lean meat like turkey or even eggs?

Chapter 6: Improving Your Metabolism

*"Calories are important. But it isn't the amount
of calories as much as the type of calories you
consume that makes a difference in terms of
how much you weigh and how healthy you
are."*
— *Dr. Mark Hyman, Author of Ultrametabolism:
The Simple Plan for Automatic Weight Loss*

L et's first define what metabolism is. While there are many variations of the term, it's medical definition is as follows:

Metabolism: The whole range of biochemical processes that occur within a living organism. Metabolism consists of anabolism (the buildup of substances) and catabolism (the breakdown of substances). The term metabolism is commonly used to refer specifically to the breakdown of food and its transformation into energy (Medical Definition of Metabolism 2016).

Most often people associate the term metabolism with weight loss and the ability for the body to break down food, but the metabolic processes in our body are complex, and, as you read, involve breaking down of substances we get from food *and* its breakdown into energy.

Most processed foods contain empty calories that don't feed our cells. Because most of us eat more empty calories than nutrient rich food, we crave more food, but we keep feeding ourselves more calorie deficient foods. Do you see why you "can't" stop eating or why you're always cravings something? So, the quality of our calories matters greatly. A woman who eats 2500 in mostly nutrient deficient food compared to a woman who eats 2500 in nutrient rich food will break down food and transform that food into energy differently. Their metabolisms will be night and day.

How about eating frequency?

I'm sure you've heard that eating more often will help boost your metabolism, but there are studies that disprove of that theory. While eating five times or more per day may not scientifically boost metabolism other studies have shown that individuals who eat fewer than three meals a day experience the perception of feeling hungrier (Campbell 2011, 157). So, aim to eat three full meals a day and snack in between meals for a total of 5 daily meals. I typically eat every 2.5 to 3 hours.

Not eating enough may cause you to gain

weight!

Are you skipping meals?

Chances are you are not eating enough, and this could be negatively impacting you and your metabolism. Most women I've talked to in the last year think that skipping meals will help with fat loss. However, the opposite is true. Not eating enough may cause you to *gain* weight! According to Lisa Young, PhD, RD, a nutritionist and adjunct professor of nutrition at New York University, not eating enough backfires. When you restrict calories too severely, your body goes into a "starvation mode". Normally, your body will use the food you eat for energy. But in starvation mode, the body uses your muscle tissue for fuel instead to conserve your fat stores. Not eating enough can actually slow down metabolism and make it harder to lose weight (Diguilio 2017). In addition, when you're hungry, you'll eat whatever is available next, and chances are you'll aim for something with little nutritional value and go overboard on your portions.

Often most people confuse thirst with

hunger, so stay hydrated!

What about food choices?

Remember, the quality of your meals counts! Aim for a mix of protein, complex carbohydrates (fruit, veggies), and good fat (polyunsaturated and monounsaturated). In addition, you need to drink a lot of water. You need at least half of your body weight worth of water every day; however, the more the better. The better hydrated you are, the less you crave. You have a sense of feeling full, so you'll eat less than you're used to when you're dehydrated. Often most people confuse *thirst* with hunger, so stay hydrated!

Fiber is key for weight loss and metabolic health!

According to the Institute of Medicine, the recommended daily intake for total fiber in women under 50 is 25 grams of fiber per day or 14 grams per 1,000 calories.

Fiber is also key in nutrition and weight loss, and according to the National Fiber Council only 10% of the population is getting enough fiber (National Fiber Council n.d.)! The National Fiber Council recommends all adults get 32 grams per day (National Fiber Council n.d.). According to the Institute of Medicine, the recommended daily intake for total fiber in women under 50 is 25 grams of fiber per day or 14 grams per 1,000 calories (Hellwig, Meyers and Otten 2006, 38, 110). Fiber also helps you feel full and curbs your hunger, so it can help you avoid the junk food and cravings too. And take note. You'll need to drink plenty of water when you up your fiber.

I've been doing lots of research on the importance of fiber in the Western diet as well as the role our gut (our large and small intestines) plays in our metabolism and health. The total bacteria in our large and small intestine is so large, it's known to scientists as its own community. Scientists commonly refer to this community as our "microbiota" (Sonnenburg and Sonnenburg 2015, 1). A diet high in fiber not only helps us digest our food more efficiently and feel full, but it plays an important role in our metabolism. How?

Our gut bacteria feed off the leftovers, particularly, complex plant polysaccharides, or dietary fiber that we normally wouldn't be able to digest (corn, for example). The microbial genes then convert this food into molecules that regulate many aspects of our biology such as the amount of inflammation in our intestines to how efficiently we store extra calories. (Sonnenburg and Sonnenburg 2015, 13,20,21).

This field of research has been popular within the last 10 years in the scientific community. While the medical community is too familiar with the bad bacteria that harm us and make us ill, we know a lot less about the trillions of "good" bacteria that line our intestinal tract in both the large and small intestine —our microbiota. These bacteria that live within us and our cells have a "symbiotic" or mutually beneficial relationship that we don't even know about!

The microbiota in your gut plays a key role in our health as well as in weight loss. In one study, obese participants with type 2 diabetes were restricted to a high fiber diet for one month. After that month those participants lost weight (Kim MS 2013, 765-775).

Conversely, what happens when lean subjects get bad gut bacteria? Dr. Jefferey Gordon, a gastroenterologist and scientist, conducts experiments on mice. In one study, Jeff's team transplanted the microbiota from obese mice into lean mice with no microbiota, and the lean mice began to gain weight with no change in diet or exercise (Sonnenburg and Sonnenburg 2015, 32).

The microbiota in your gut plays a key role

in our health as well as in weight loss.

Many other studies have found that leaner and healthier mice and human populations have a diverse "microbiota" (Denjean 2013). Additionally, scientists have noted that leaner populations with richer and more diverse gut bacteria can also burn fat at higher rates (Denjean 2013).

When comparing gut bacteria in obese individuals and subjects to lean individuals and subjects, the gut bacteria in obese populations are a lot less diverse. And to take it a bit further, or international, when comparing a Western Individual's gut bacteria to those of an individual in third world countries, we see less diverse microbiota in our guts than those of our third world counterparts (Sonnenburg and Sonnenburg 2015, 1).

This could be because the Western diet has gotten so processed and away from whole foods, whereas our third world neighbors may still eat more traditional and local whole foods.

In addition to the metabolic benefits of eating more fiber, scientists are also studying how our microbiota communicates with our central nervous system and hormones not only to work in our favor with weight loss, but in even regulating our moods (Farmer, Randall and Aziz 2014, 2981–2988) and (Denjean 2013). So, there are plenty of reasons to enjoy fiber throughout the day!

Another study found that a particular strain of gut bacteria called Akkermansia Muciniphila worked in the microbiota to help lose fat *and* improve mood in lean populations (Denjean 2013). So, there is proof that certain gut bacteria will help aid in the fat loss process.

As cool as this research sounds, the research is still in its infancy, and like the Human Genome Project, there is also a Human Microbiome Project to sequence all the genes in the human microbiota and look for correlations between microbiome changes and health changes (NIH, National Institutes of Health n.d.). There are new studies every day on how our microbiota impacts our health and wellness and how certain strands either increase or reduce inflammation.

And just in case you were wondering…

What should you eat to improve the health of your gut bacteria?

Yes, a diet rich in fiber, whether in the

form of complex carbs and grains like

brown-rice, quinoa, and super-grains and

fruits and vegetables, helps feed our gut

bacteria, which in turn help us boost our

metabolism.

According to the UBiome Blog, polyphenol-rich foods helps increase Akkermansia Muciniphila in the gut. And polyphenols can be found in many fruits especially cranberries, blueberries, and blackberries (but remember to go organic)!

Administration of polyphenol to obese mice has shown to reduce the detrimental effects of obesity and increase Akkermansia abundance. Cranberries contain Proanthocyanidins (PAC), a polyphenol, which has a prebiotic effect on Akkermansia. (Taylor 2016)

Polyphenols are chemicals that act as antioxidants to protect the body against damage (MedicineNet.com 2017). As you can see there is more to fiber than meets the eye and curiosity! Yes, a diet rich in fiber, whether in the form of complex carbs and grains like brown-rice, quinoa, and super-grains and fruits and vegetables, helps feed our gut bacteria, which in turn help us boost our metabolism. You'll find a list of polyphenol rich foods where you download your workbook.

In summary, studies have shown that our gut bacteria genes work within our metabolic processes to help us lose fat, stabilize our blood sugar levels, and our hormones involved with mood, and even help in reducing inflammation in the body. Who knew fiber could play a strong role in the health of the good bacteria that reside in our gut and help us lose weight and regulate our metabolism and mood!

Remember, most processed foods we are eating give us empty calories that don't provide us with enough energy! These foods and snacks don't compare to the energy we get from whole fresh food (fruits, veggies and anything living). We are not eating enough live, good energy and underfeeding our gut bacteria, which help us with our metabolism!

If you aren't already tracking your fiber daily, I recommend you begin to. Your food labels include the percent daily value of fiber and the grams of fiber. Whenever you're hungry and are looking for a good snack, opt for something high in protein and high in fiber. Remember, if you're eating from a box, it's "man-made" food. If you can help it, opt for living whole food! I've included a sample meal plan achieving 25 grams of fiber for a woman under 50 in the appendix of this book! If you'd like to see a more comprehensive list of fiber found in grains, fruits and veggies, you can get that where you'll get your downloadable workbook!

Think deeply about your health and eating habits, whatever you're doing is either prolonging or shortening your existence, so always work on improving your nutrition and health habits! I like to think of it just like the actor William Hurt, who plays Dr. George Millican on the British Sci-Fi Drama TV series Humans:

> *"If you're not worried about dying, you're not really living. You're just existing."*

Are you living today or just existing?

Chapter 7: Mindset and Passion Matter

"The only way that we can live, is if we grow.
The only way that we can grow is if we change.
The only way that we can change is if we learn.
The only way we can learn is if we are exposed.
And the only way that we can become exposed
is if we throw ourselves out into the open. Do it.
Throw yourself."

— *C. JoyBell C., Author and Inspirational Figure*

Wow! How's this quote for an 'ah ha!' My goal is that you find the tips and tools to grow from reading this book and completing your written exercises. Where your mind and focus go, your energy will flow! As you can see, what you believe about food, fitness, and yourself sometimes, are not always positive or correct! Maintaining a positive mindset and working on your passions will take you a long way in improving your overall health, fitness, and life.

To maintain a positive mindset, you need to surround yourself with people who are positive. I recently shared a video on Facebook about cleaning up your social media feed. Remove anyone spewing negativity on your social media feed. Remove the negative news sources, negative people, and negative pages. You don't want anything that's not positive to dominate or pop up on your feed.

Read positive books. Determine that you won't stand for anything negative. It's tough to clear the negative clutter from your daily thoughts. But once you surround yourself with positive people and surround yourself with positive resources; books, TV programs, web sites, and your social media feeds, it will help you maintain a positive mindset.

Have you ever considered what your life's purpose was?

Why did God choose you to live here on this earth at this particular moment in time? I like to believe that each one of us is placed here to accomplish our own individual mission that's part of a larger movement, but the clutter and lack of belief within ourselves often keeps us away from finding that purpose and making a huge impact on the lives of others. And this mission, once you realize what it is, will drive you to act and be decisive. Your newfound purpose will help take your value and importance to the next level, and you'll find yourself wanting to improve your health more to fulfill that mission. **Take out your workbook and give some thought to what your mission is.**

Ask yourself:

- What do I stand for?
- What am I passionate about?
- How do I enjoy helping others?
- Who do I enjoy helping the most?

If you're having some challenges thinking of your passions, what three things can you never give up doing to stay in your happy place?

For me it's inspiring, singing, and creating content, books, and helpful tools for women who need a nudge to *Defeat It!*

Can you think of your three passions now? Determine now that your mission in life is greater. Write your passions down now!

My Passions

1) _____
2) _____
3) _____

What Can You Do?

I have a mantra. It's this:

"What can I do now?"

Get used to asking yourself that question! Focus on what you CAN do. Never focus on what you can't do at any given moment. In fact, remove the words "I'll try" and "I can't" from your vocabulary. Any time I feel in a slump or I feel discouraged, I ask myself what can I do this very moment to _____. What can I do now?

What can *you* do now (today) to live your healthiest? It may be finish reading this book and completing the exercises.

If I'm thinking about building my business, I ask myself, "What can I do now to build my business?" If I'm thinking about becoming a better mom, I ask myself, "What can I do now to help me be a better mom?" If I'm feeling like I'm slacking at any point in my fitness, and yes that does happen from time to time, I ask myself, "What can I do now to improve my energy and motivation?"

Always focus on what you CAN do and never on what you can't. When you continue to place your focus on inability, you'll feel incapable, and defeated. You'll be reluctant to begin anything when you focus on inability, but when you find yourself looking towards and focusing on what you can do and what's possible, you'll start to make things happen!

Remember, defeat is only temporary, and temporary defeat is not failure! Analyze temporary defeat and see how you can use it to your advantage!

Remember, defeat is only temporary, and temporary defeat is not failure! Analyze temporary defeat and see how you can use it to your advantage! Start looking at all the events that happen in your life as opportunities for you to learn and grow into the person God wants you to be. It's not about the big goal. Ultimately, it's not about the body, the money, or the job you want. It's about *who* you become in the process. For instance, if you got plastic surgery without working on your insecurities, you'd have the body you always wanted but you'd still have all your insecurities. *Who* you become in the process is worth more than the end goal!

Who you become in the process is worth

more than the end goal!

What "negative" things have happened to you recently? How can you reframe those experiences and use them as an opportunity for growth or learning a lesson?

_____

_____

_____

_____

_____

_____

_____

_____

_____

_____

They say that you're the average of the five closest people you hang out with, so vet your friends, both online and offline, and fill your life with positivity. This will go a very long way. Who are you hanging out with the most now? Do you need more positive friends?

List your closest friends below.

1) _____

2) _____

3) _____

4) _____

5) _____

You may find that you may need to stop hanging out so much with a few friends. That's ok. You will set an example for others by working on you.

...working on your mindset is a daily work

in progress.

Implementing these few tips will help you maintain a positive mindset, but working on your mindset is a *daily* work in progress. Just like it will take some effort on your end to change your eating and exercising habits, it will take effort for you to work on your mindset. Developing a positive mindset takes years to do just like becoming a super fit woman will take you some time, but the many small steps added over time will get you to your goals and shape you into the amazing person that's growing in you. Rewiring your mind is the same process. Just keep at it. And work on your mind even more than you work on your body!

Chapter 8: Motivation Strategies To WIN

"Lack of emotion causes lack of progress and lack of motivation."

– Tony Robbins, World-renowned author, speaker and peak performance strategist

Motivation is something that's very personal and each of us have different things that help us motivate to act. Motivation can come from something within us or external forces like people, friends, and family. When it comes from something that wells up from within us, it's called intrinsic motivation, and if it's something that we get from external sources, it's called extrinsic motivation. We all have different motivators both intrinsic and extrinsic.

So how can you motivate yourself when you're feeling down or when you want to give up? I believe motivation boils down to finding your *why* and purpose in life. This is the reason we just did the exercise on finding your passions. (If you need to go back and do it, do it now!)

But when it comes to your fitness, ask yourself:

- Why is it that you really want to be in better shape?
- Why do you want to lose the weight?
- Why do you want to eat healthier?

- What problem will getting in better shape, becoming healthier, or dropping the extra weight solve for you?
- Will your goal help you build more confidence?
- Will your goal help you feel more energized and productive?
- Will it solve a deeper pain that you quite haven't scratched the surface of just yet?

When you start getting "grit" or become motivated to tackle a challenge, you need to have a strong, meaningful, and personal WHY. It can't be something superficial like, "I want to look good for me." Or "I want to look good to impress someone." It must be something that's tied to a deep-rooted *emotion*, whether it's self-love, self-esteem, a crazy life-changing event, something like a divorce, or something that has deep roots or a deep gut-feeling.

Think about your why. Within your workbook, list 10-20 reasons why you want to get fit now. I've provided 10 lines below, but you can add more in your workbook.

Brainstorm and circle the top three reasons why you want to get fit. Tie that with a deep-seated emotion or fear. Remember, your why must be strong and unique to YOU. When your why is strong, you'll find that it'll be easier to get motivated when you don't want to get up to go to the gym or you don't want to work out at home.

I want to get fit and lose/gain _____ pounds because:

1) _____

2) _____

3) _____

4) _____

5) _____

6) _____

7) _____

8) _____

9) _____

10) _____

Again, make your reasons super personal and unique to you. What things or people motivate you? Is your motivation intrinsic or something that comes from within? Maybe you have a competitive spark within you that helps motivate you. Or maybe you're extrinsically motivated by your children, your siblings, or by being a role model.

List five things that motivate you:

1) _____

2) _____

3) _____

4) _____

5) _____

List five people who motivate you that you can either talk to you when you're in the dumps or that'll help encourage you. Keep this list always so that whenever you're depressed or unmotivated, you can reach out to one of these people.

1) _____

2) _____

3) _____

4) _____

5) _____

Make It Personal And Set A Deadline

Now that you know your WHY, what's your specific fitness goal over the next three months? For instance, "I want to lose 20 lbs. in three months."

Now add your deeper emotions into the reason you want to achieve this goal. What do you want to achieve by getting fit? See this as an example:

"I want to lose 20 lbs. in the next three months because it will help me feel better about myself and be less self-conscious at work when conducting presentations. Dropping the weight will help me become more secure in my personal relationships and will help me be less insecure and more confident."

See how this super personal statement is rooted in deeper issues in the person's life? Make your reason personal!

They say goals are dreams with a deadline! And the above reasons will help fuel your goals. You've written things you intend to do, but take it further and like the example above, write a brief paragraph summarizing your why and your intention to get fit. Remember, set a deadline by which you want to achieve this goal and put it in your calendar with checkpoint reminders!

Write your statement of intention and set your date:

_____

_____

_____

_____

_____

_____

_____

_____

Date to Reach Goal:

_____

Now, think about reaching your goal. For you to reach your goal, who is the person that you need to become? What qualities do you need to have? Don't worry if you exhibit those qualities now or later. You will become who you set yourself out to become! Write it down. Write down the person that you need to become.

I need to become someone who (list traits):

_____

_____

_____

_____

_____

_____

_____

What habits do you need to remove and what habits do you need to add in your life to achieve that goal?

The habits I need to change are:

    1) _____

    2) _____

    3) _____

Anticipate how you can replace those habits. Write down at least 3 things you can to do replace your habits.

I can replace those habits by:

    1) _____

    2) _____

    3) _____

Think about the things that need to happen now and three months from now to achieve your goal. List five things that need to happen, between now and three months from now for you to make progress on your goal. Think about six months in the future. What else needs to happen?

Five Things That Need to Happen Within 3 Months

1) _____

2) _____

3) _____

4) _____

5) _____

Three Additional Things That Need to Happen Within 6 Months

1) _____

2) _____

3) _____

If you can think of any challenges that you need to overcome, think about those challenges in advance. Brainstorm and list all the challenges that are possible. And then think about ways that you could overcome those challenges.

Challenges I Anticipate

1) _____

2) _____

3) _____

How I Plan to Overcome Those Challenges

1) _____

2) _____

3) _____

Visualize your success.

How will you feel after having reached your goal?

_____

_____

_____

_____

_____

_____

_____

How will the quality of life change for the better once you've reached that first big milestone?

_____

_____

_____

_____

_____

_____

_____

_____

Chapter 9: Overcoming Negative Emotions

"Feelings are something you have; not something you are."

— Shannon L. Alder, Inspirational Author

As a woman, it's challenging to overcome your emotions, particularly when you're pregnant. One of my lowest points in life came as a 36-year-old pregnant woman in her first trimester. The path that lead me to gaining 13 pounds in about a month was a spiraling, negative mindset.

Yes. You heard me correctly. After all this positive talk and years of building my positive mindset, I went backwards. And even after my defining moment in that car accident the summer of 2012, I went back to negative thinking after I got pregnant with my third child in my late 30s. This is expected in any life journey — fitness related or not. It's okay to sit in a funk as long as you get back up again and recognize that defeat is only temporary!

I've grown into this healthy positive-minded person over time. So, being positive isn't a complete "on" and "off" switch, though once you're more of a positive person, you can more easily control those negative thoughts and send them to H.E...double hockey sticks – where they come from! It's takes practice.

It's okay to sit in a funk as long as you get

back up again and recognize that defeat is

only temporary!

But if you're working on your positivity and mindset, how do you snap yourself out of a negative down-spiral or those nagging thoughts?

You just begin to monitor your thoughts. Filter them. And write them down in a journal if it helps. If the thoughts are not serving you to become a better version of who you were yesterday, toss them out and replace them with the opposite, healthier emotion. Write down the opposite, healthy, and positive emotion in your journal. Practice filtering them with your spouse or a good friend too.

It may sound easier said than done, but you can start filling your mind with more positive than negative, and then you will begin to catch the bad thoughts more often.

As mentioned earlier in the book, start vetting through what you watch (TV, music, social media) etc. What and *who* you surround yourself with will play a big part in your daily set of emotions. Make it a point to not read negative news, delete negative friends from your social media feeds (or unfollow). Start listening to positive music. Find your local Christian radio station and decide to only listen to positive and uplifting music. Find positive role models to hang around with, whether that be online or in person (or both).

Another thing that will help is to stop comparing yourself to others. Just as you read in the beginning of this book; stop feeling defeated, everyone else is on a different path and journey. Focus and work towards becoming a better version of who you were yesterday every single day.

Faith is a huge part of my journey. I pray often and I work on building my relationship with God. I am not the best at it, but I work towards it. Prayer helps me. I highly recommend that you try prayer, and that you surround yourself with others who believe in a greater power, who believe in God, and begin attending and serving in your local church. Attending services will help you continue to self-reflect and fine-tune your emotions and actions.

Once you find a good church home and are comfortable, begin serving. The sooner you do this the better! Serving in my local church has empowered me to share my love of life and God to help give others hope.

Fight to remain positive, and look to our creator for wisdom and signs. They are there if you ask for them, and even if you don't!

I'd like to share a few of my favorite Bible verses with you. These are from the King James Version (KJV):

By Dali Burgado, CPT

I can do all things through Christ which strengtheneth me.

Philippians 4:13

Ask and it shall be given you; seek and ye shall find; knock, and it shall be opened unto you.

Matthew 7:7

Be careful for nothing; but in every thing by prayer and supplication with thanksgiving let your requests be made known unto God. And the peace of God, which passeth all understanding, shall keep your hearts and minds through Christ Jesus.

Philippians 4:6-7

Have not I commanded thee? Be strong and of a good courage; be not afraid, neither be thou dismayed: for the Lord thy God is with thee whithersoever thou goest.

Joshua 1:9

Therefore do not worry about tomorrow, for tomorrow will worry about itself. Each day has enough trouble of its own.

Matthew 6:34

By Dali Burgado, CPT

It shall be health to thy navel, and marrow to thy bones.

Proverbs 3:8

Express Your Emotions

Expressing myself has not been easy for me, but this is another area where I've grown tremendously over the years. This was hard for me especially because growing up, my mother had no serious talks or discussions with me. My father never did either. Even my 4 older siblings never did. I would bottle everything up, and adapted it as the norm.

If you're anything like me, a "bottler of emotions", you'll find that it's hard to even talk with those whom you're closest to, like your spouse, your children, or anyone for that matter, especially if you're a private person.

But whenever you're feeling low, you always need to have at least one person, whether it's someone close to you, or maybe somebody from church or a friend who won't judge you to talk to so you can get those negative emotions out, or just whatever it is that you're feeling. It's very important to communicate that, to let it out. If you need to cry, let it out. Especially when you're pregnant you'll find that you're very emotional and you're easier to cry, so just let it out.

After child-birth, you will likely experience post-partum depression. And that's normal. Allow yourself the time to cry, vent, or talk to someone. I firmly believe that the healthier you eat, the less depressed you feel. Remember the gut bacteria and mood studies! I felt the depression after my first two pregnancies but have kept my sanity after the third. I don't feel that same depression after my third pregnancy. It's been my healthiest time, and I don't think it is coincidental. Whether you really feel or acknowledge the depression, you need an outlet. Exercise, diet, friends, and professionals can help you cope with any kind of depression, even post-partum.

Love Your Body at Every Stage!

With centuries and years of misogynistic views of women, it's no wonder women struggle with body image and self-confidence. I grew up in the 80s and 90s, but at the start of the 90s I remember it was just a plastic surgery craze. Plastic surgery had become popular then, and it was difficult for me as a developing teenager to watch certain shows, or commercials, or listen to radio commercials and ads that pushed changing and rearranging your body, especially with breast implants.

I have never been heavily endowed up there, so the plastic surgery marketing was annoying to me. I was always happy with myself, but more importantly with my spirit. But when I looked at my reflection in the mirror and my small top, I *had to* always tell myself I was beautiful, and that I was perfect the way I was because I didn't want to get sucked into that negativity marketing bombardment.

So, if you need to limit certain TV shows that portray women as objects, or are just filled with plastic, don't watch those shows. Remove those types of shows from your watch list, because it's not going to be healthy for your self-confidence or your self-esteem.

> Look at yourself in the mirror every day. As long as you grow as an individual, as a woman, and you're working towards building the body that you want, love it no matter what stage you are in.

Look at yourself in the mirror every day. As long as you grow as an individual, as a woman, and you're working towards building the body that you want, love it no matter what stage you are in. Love where you are. Love what you see in the mirror right now.

Tell yourself daily that you are beautiful, you are unique, and you are loved. You were created for a purpose.

God doesn't make mistakes, and he put you on this earth for a reason. So, *own your beauty*. Own your uniqueness. Remove any negative people, negative TV shows, imagery, and things like that from your daily experience. I know that truly helped me out as a teenager who was starting to build self-confidence. Tell yourself, "I am enough."

Tell yourself daily that you are beautiful,

you are unique, and you are loved. You

were created for a purpose.

And remember this. You *are* enough! I hope you feel inspired so far! Read on to discover the stories of other women who've *Defeated their "It".* Here's to overcoming and defeating your it!

Chapter 10: Fitspirational Interviews

The following chapter includes a series of interviews with four women who decided to *Defeat It!* and make positive changes in their health and fitness. These women lost at least 20 lbs. or more within three months by changing their physical activity levels and diet.

Each of these women faced fears, challenges, and obstacles. However, they each managed to *Defeat It!*

In their interviews, I ask them:

- How they overcame these challenges and fears in their fitness journey
- What motivated them to begin the journey in the first place
- What motivated them throughout the journey
- How the journey changed each of them in the process

I hope you find inspiration in each of their stories and take some of their experiences and advice on how to defeat your own "it"!

Interview with Ronnie Dent

Ronnie is a thirty-something working mom of two children under the age of five, a teacher, wife, and church volunteer.

R onnie defeated negative body image and excuses. Ronnie lost 25 lbs.

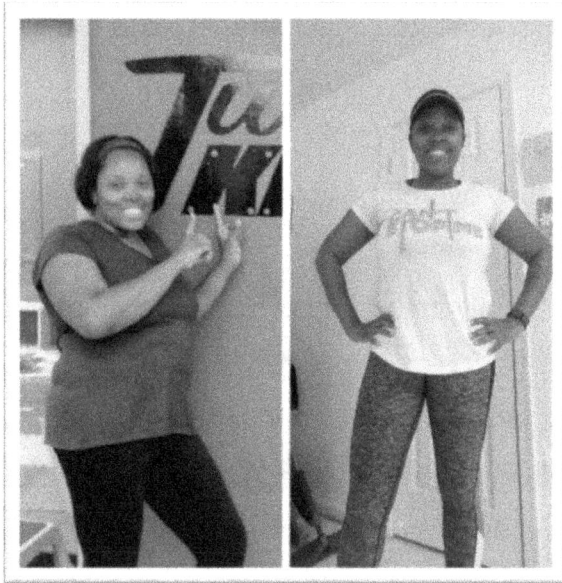

BEFORE   **AFTER**

Dali: Today I'm here with Ronnie Dent. Ronnie's lost about 25 pounds in her fitness journey. Ronnie, what motivated you to begin your journey? What was that one defining moment for you?

Ronnie: In June of 2016 I was finishing up physical therapy on my back. After I had my son Noah, I started to have bad lower back pain. I thought it was from the epidural because that can cause back pain. But it lasted for a long time until he was one.

No medicine worked, and I finally ended up having an MRI. The doctor suggested that I could probably fix it with physical therapy or else I would need surgery. So, I started physical therapy. After the physical therapy was done, I was determined to get back into the gym and start working out so I wouldn't have any major health issues.

Dali: So, it was the back pain and the therapy that was your defining moments and motivated you to take action?

Ronnie: Yes. Because the pain was very severe. Once I had the MRI the issue shook me up. I didn't want to have to deal with that pain. I told myself once I saw the physical therapist I would do whatever they said to get my health back in order.

Dali: So, before you started your journey what emotions or feelings did you have that encouraged you to get going?

Ronnie: I have two children, I'm married, I work, and juggling all that wears you out. And I was exhausted all the time. It was little things like going up and down the stairs and doing the laundry that would fatigue me. It really bothered me that I couldn't get through simple daily activities without being out of breath or being exhausted.

I was always exhausted throughout the day. Trying to juggle everything really took a toll on me. I didn't want to continue doing the things I was doing and get older and have all these major health issues.

I also wanted to set a good example for my children. Growing up, I wasn't very active or exercised. I wanted my children to know that exercise is something you should do daily not because you are trying to lose weight but that is something you should do regularly.

I wanted that especially for my daughter because I struggled with low self-esteem as a teenager. I don't want her to struggle with poor body image. I want her to be confident starting now. I don't want her to deal with yo-yo dieting or worrying about what she looks like. I want to show her that living a healthy active lifestyle is something that you should do.

It starts from when you're small. You pick up all these habits and learn what's around you.

Dali: It's awesome to use your kids as motivation.

Ronnie: They love working out with me!

Dali: Did you have any fears or worries as you started your journey?

Ronnie: The biggest thing for me was balancing it all and having that consistency. I think when you first start you can do too much too soon. For me, I knew it was something I didn't want to do temporarily and stop in three months. I knew this was something I wanted to make a habit and continue to do this 10 years from now, so I look for a lot of things that have longevity to it and not a fad or get quick results. I wanted to do something to be consistent with it. So, the big thing and concern was balance since I'm married with two children.

Dali: How did you manage to find that balance?

Ronnie: I came up with a plan. I started running years ago and picked it up again. I loved it.

I try to limit a lot of excuses. One of them is having kids. "Oh, I can't work out because I have kids. And what am I going to do with them." So, I try to find ways to get my kids involved. Because I'm a teacher, I have the summers off, and they are home with me. Instead of making the excuse that I can't go for a run because the kids are with me, I found some tracks in the area, and I asked people I knew for recommendations. I found tracks with playgrounds. While I ran, the kids played in the playground. And sometimes my kids would run laps or the kids would ride their bikes as I would run. I would find things like that to eliminate excuses.

And, if I go to the gym, I'd take them with me. They got excited about going to the gym with me. I got rid of those excuses and that allowed me to keep working out.

Dali: I love that idea. Finding a park with trails!

Ronnie: Another thing I would do is schedule my workouts in my calendar and then send an invite to my husband to remind him that I'm going to the gym today and a reminder would pop up on both our phones, so he knew I was going to the gym at whatever time. And it would help him to support me with my goals. It's helpful for me too because I can plan it and I also put what class I'm taking or what I'm going to do if I'm going to run. It puts it in my mind and holds me accountable!

I also pack my gym bag at night so it's ready. And that's another excuse I could get rid of (not having my gym bag ready). I have the bag in my car, and I'm ready to go.

Dali: Did you find other unexpected challenges by being more active? Any challenges with your beliefs?

Ronnie: I hit a plateau. One of the things I think I faced as I increased my activity was a plateau where I'd stop losing weight. So, I had to change what I was doing. I added different things like new classes and new ways to work out. I started paying more attention more to what I was eating too.

Also, a few months ago, things got hard at work and home, and that was a challenge. But I found that the working out helped me push through those different challenges because it gave me a lot of endurance when I didn't feel like working out or something became difficult, it gave me something to focus on.

Dali: Yes. That's huge. The stress-relieving aspect of working out and looking forward to it because of the challenges you face outside of the gym.

Ronnie: Right. Yes. That helped me push through other situations because I knew I could do it. It's something that's very fulfilling. When you don't feel like you can do it and feel like you're about to give up and you actually do it. And that helped me. I realize I am a lot stronger than I think I am.

Dali: Who did you become in the journey as you started working out and began eating better and doing different things? Look at yourself back then and now. Who did you become?

Ronnie: I'm definitely more confident. I'm okay with the way I look and what I can do. I think being able to set a goal and reach it has been very encouraging. And I realize I'm a lot stronger than I thought I was.

It's very encouraging to be able to pick up the weights and think, "Oh this is easy." Where before I thought, I was going to die. So, it's very encouraging to set a goal and to reach it and to be able to set more goals.

I've learned to accept my body and the way I look. I don't compare myself to others like I did before.

Dali: That's big! Yes. Women do that a lot and even men (they size themselves up at the gym).

Ronnie: I've learned to accept my body for what it is. I know what I'm capable of, but I'm not afraid to try something new. The biggest thing is that confidence.

Dali: Was there anything else that kept you motivated in your journey?

Ronnie: Yes. Seeing my kids watch me and seeing how excited they were to help me along the journey whether it was going for walks or going to the gym. Also, watching other people in my family who are overweight and being able to encourage them and see them watch me reach my goals has been encouraging. To change the atmosphere in my family has been very motivating!

For me it wasn't only the physical weight but there was a lot of emotional weight for a long time. That has been very motivating as well. As I drop the pounds I also let go of other emotional things as well that I've struggled with over the years, for instance, low self-esteem.

Dali: Expand a little bit more on the emotional weight.

Ronnie: I think growing up I was bullied, and I struggled with my weight as a teenager. Girls can be mean, and boys can be mean too. So, I dealt a lot with that. I didn't like who I was. I compared myself to a lot of people. And it took me a long time to be okay with who I am.

Now, I'm okay with what I look like and the way my body looks. I know who I am and what I'm capable of. And that's ok. I've learned to let go of what people think and expect of me. Going through this journey, I know who I am and what I'm doing. There is a great peace in that. That for me, has been instrumental. That not only have I lost a lot of physical weight but just letting go of what others think of me or expect of me and being comfortable in who I am.

Dali: Did you use any other motivational tools like an accountability partner, a trainer, or fun visuals?

Ronnie: Not really. But I have friends that would text me and say, "Hey, are you going to the gym today?" I have friends who go to the same classes. So, I have friends that check in with me.

Dali: How much did that motivate you or help you stay consistent?

Ronnie: It helps because when you go the gym and people say, "Hey, I missed you at the gym today," sometimes that makes you feel bad. And wow, people notice when I'm not here. And another thing is I would always buy more workout clothes as I lost weight. I find shirts with quirky sayings like, "Princess," or "Awesomeness" with the letters "me" highlighted. Recently, I bought a shirt that says, "can't stop me." Things like that help me keep going. I also have a tumbler that says, "There is no change without a challenge." I always look at that cup and it helps me to keep going. If you want change, you must be willing to change. That's going to be difficult, but if you want to make something happen, you must be willing to do it. I thought about hanging a little bikini but I haven't yet.

Dali: I love the t-shirts. I enjoy that too. Overall, what would you say changed about you as a mom, wife, or woman after your transformation?

Ronnie: The balance. I'm more balanced and less stressed. Going to the gym is my "me time." So, between work and coming home, I have that time to destress and unwind and deal with everything else I have going on in life. Exercising is now something that I need to do. It's not an option, and it's now a habit. The more I take care of myself, the more I can take care of other things in my life.

Dali: Thank you. I'm sure the ladies reading this will be very inspired by this.

By Dali Burgado, CPT

Interview with Melanie Yost

50-Year-Old Mother of 1, Wife and Business Owner

Melanie defeated fear of dieting and comparing herself to others. Melanie lost her first 20 lbs. and then, within a year lost 50 lbs.

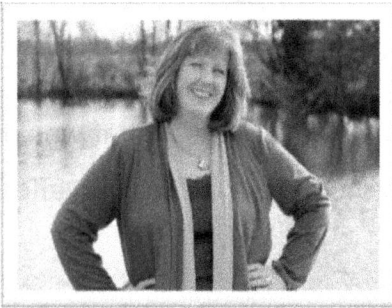

BEFORE

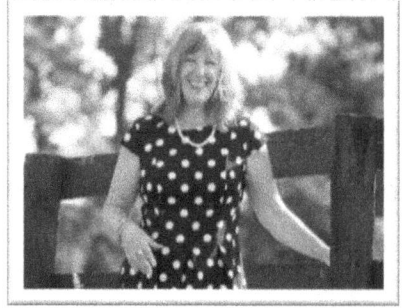

AFTER

Dali: Melanie, what motivated you to begin your journey? What was that moment or that experience that helped you get going?

Melanie: What got me really motivated to start exercising was my mom had a significant health crisis. And she was in the hospital. Looking back, she was really ill. I had gained a lot of weight. I was tired, and I wasn't exercising. I wasn't doing anything. My mother was having issues with her knees and her mobility. I could see my future, and I did not want to be immobile.

I joined a Cross Fit Gym and then started exercising, and that helped me manage the anxiety I was going through as I was helping my mom. My daughter was transitioning to middle school, I was taking care of my mom, and I was running my business. I was so stressed out, so it helped me manage that stress. That's what got me off the couch and into the gym.

Dali: What feelings did you have before you started? What emotions did you feel before getting started or those first few days of your fitness journey?

Melanie: Before getting started, I was stressed. That whole year, it was the year I joke that I limped to the finish line. So, leading up to that moment was all stress. The first few days of working out, my first workout was all of 5 minutes, I just felt like I was going to die. It was hard, and I thought to myself a lot, "What are you thinking?"

Interestingly enough, that's also what kept me going back. I've never loved exercise, period. And that's one of the things I love about the gym I go to. I love seeing a workout and thinking that's just crazy. I think there is no way I can do that. And then I do it. And then I have this feeling that if I can do that, I can do anything. That was super empowering in those first few months. If I can finish this exercise. Sometimes with every rep, I was thinking "ok…don't die." And I remember I was running, and I hate running, and I was thinking if I can do this, if I can finish this workout everything else I have today will be easy. So, that's what kept me going.

Dali: Did you have any fears in the beginning or maybe, like in the second week or beyond? Was there anything that was frightening about what you were doing, or working out, or how you felt about working out?

Melanie: I can't say. Some of the workouts were scary, but they were all scalable. Like a hand-stand push up. I was like there's no way, but everything is scalable. So, any fears I had about how hard something was ended up being okay because I was able to do a modified version of the workout.

Now, I'm going to tell you since it was a journey, I started working out, and I lost weight, but then I gained it. So, like, 15 months after I started the gym, I did a paleo diet challenge.

And that's really when I lost a lot of weight that I've kept off. So, it was the exercise and changing my diet because what I found was I was still managing my emotions through a crappy diet, so no matter how much I was exercising the weight wasn't coming off. It had to go hand-in-hand. So, my big fears were around changing my diet, because I remember when I first started at the gym, the owner said, "Hey. What do you think about doing the Paleo diet?" And I was like, "No because I've never met a bread I didn't like, sugar is my drug of choice, and if a little cheese is good, more is better!" And I had to give all that up!

And so, it was, like, 15 months later and I finally was in the right mindset to make changes in my diet. I had to do something because my joints were aching, and I just didn't feel well. It was getting harder to work out. And I even gained the weight back that I had initially lost. And so, it was an eight-week challenge. It was very, very strict paleo, and then within the eight-week challenge, I lost probably 20 pounds.

And then I went on, and I'm still eating probably 80% to 90% Paleo, so I'm not super strict because I never want to feel deprived. I cut it off, but I ended up losing over 50 pounds overall.

Dali: That's awesome.

Melanie: So yeah, then I was scared to death to give up sugar, grains, and dairy (as is the case with the Paleo diet).

Dali: So, when you first started that diet, were you all-in or did it take you time to settle into it?

Melanie: I was all-in. In fact, I signed up for the challenge and had to do check-ins and we had to do workouts and all of that. And then Brian (my husband) just did it with me. But I was all-in. I did not cheat, not once. A lot of people who were doing it cheated. I did not cheat, not once.

It was eight weeks, and even the last week of the challenge and we went to an Octoberfest at my husband's parent's house, like his family is all food-centered, and they all got together. And there was this delicious food spread. They made homemade soft pretzels, and they were baking in the oven. And I was like, "You're killing me," but what I found was once I broke some habits the cravings went away. And now when I eat stuff that I don't normally eat, periodically I'll have pizza or a cheeseburger with the bun, when I do that, I don't feel good. My joints ache and my stomach gets upset.

Dali: How difficult was it going all in?

Melanie: It was a challenge we started dropping out things 2 weeks before. So, we eased into it so that once the challenge started we were all in. And by the time the challenge started, it was ok. And I was just so ready, that it really wasn't that hard.

Dali: That's a cool strategy—dropping things gradually during the 2 weeks. Did that help?

Melanie: Yes, it did help. I had to wrap my mind around it first though because sugar is my drug of choice, and that was the last thing that I completely dropped. I cut way back before the challenge, but when the challenge started, I had none.

Dali: Beyond the Paleo diet was there an obstacle or challenge you had to overcome?

Melanie: In this whole journey, I've gotten injured a couple times. I've hurt my hips a few times and hurt my shoulder, so I had to really start to listen to my body. I'm going on 50 in March this year, and so I really need to listen more to my body. In the Cross Fit environment, especially, it can be very tempting to overdo it because you see these people going hard. They may be your age or a lot younger than you, and they're throwing around ridiculous amounts of weights and just doing amazing things.

There can be this push that you're "sandbagging it" or you're slacking. But because I'm older now, I need to listen to my body. Three times a week is really the max that I can do a Cross Fit workout. Even though in Cross Fit they encourage you to workout 5-6 times a week, 3 times a week at that level of intensity is what *my* body can handle. And even then, sometimes 3 times is too much for me. I had to learn to listen to my body.

Dali: When was that first time where you remember feeling something and saying, "Hey, I think I'm listening to my body now."?

Melanie: Well, after my first injury. When I hurt my hip, I didn't want to quit going to the gym, but I also didn't want to injure myself again. So, I warm up well beforehand, and I stretch out well afterwards. So, yeah. It was after my first injury, and I was like, "I've got to be able to function. I'm not 20, and I don't bounce back like I did when I was 20, so I really need to be smart about this."

Dali: You pointed out something else that I think is important too. When you see other people doing amazing things at the gym you either feel inadequate or like you said that you're not pushing enough, and you compare yourself to others.

Melanie: You do. We do that all the time. We compare ourselves. A lot of the workouts are done for time, so it's do 5 rounds of these things for time. There are people in there that just whip through it and are done super quickly. And when you're constantly the last person to get done, it can really mess with you. One of my very first workouts – I still have a picture of it on my phone – it was horrible. Like the class was done and the next class had started, and I was still going.

My coach was there with me cheering me on. It was Burpees and Kettlebells. It was awful. It was terrible that the class was done, the people were packed up and gone, and the next class had started, and still I am there with the Kettlebell and doing Burpees. It was horrible. That was definitely one of those workouts that when I finished, I said, "If I can do that, then anything else I do today is going to be easy."

Dali: I think you point out 2 great lessons. First, listen to your body. And second, don't compare yourself to anyone else.

Melanie: Exactly. The other thing I learned when lifting weights, to me it's not so much how much I lift but whatever amount I lift, I'm going to lift with good form because that's how I got hurt in the first place.

I was not lifting with the proper form, and that's how I hurt my hip. I went back and stripped the bar, and I and started super light. That's where then if you're competitive at all then you start to mess with yourself. I'm competitive with myself, and if I think I'm slacking off I give myself a hard time. So here I am doing back squats with a stripped-down bar, and people are doing crazy numbers. And you think you're slacking, but it's what I needed to get my form correct. As soon as my form was correct, I could add weight, and now I stop as soon as my form starts to go. But now I'm getting back up there in my numbers, but good form is what's most important for me.

So, it's listening to my body, leaving my ego at the door, and making sure I'm doing what I need to do with good form.

Dali: In your fitness journey who would you say you became in the process? Compare yourself before Cross Fit until now. What's changed?

Melanie: I think the biggest thing is that I feel comfortable in my body so when you start exercising and you start pushing your body to, sometimes, its limits then you know what things it can and cannot do, and you get more comfortable in it. And I felt more empowered. And that was important to me. It was super empowering when I started exercising. This is the longest I've exercised consistently, ever. So, I feel empowered to do things.

I really like the functional fitness – pushups, pullups, and things that are functional. As much as I hate burpees, the ability to get up from the floor quickly is important. So, I'm much empowered, and I'm just more comfortable in my skin.

Dali: Can you think of what kept you motivated when things got tough with the diet or the workouts?

Melanie: The feeling of being pain-free. The thing with the diet is it's not that hard to follow because when I eat something I don't normally eat, I feel terrible. My joints hurt, and I physically don't feel well. Like over the holidays, I ate way more sugar and bread than I'm used to, and everything hurt. I was congested. I was fuzzy-headed. I've been doing Paleo for over 3 years now, so I feel it physically, and I'm very aware of that.

For me, it's easier to eat Paleo. For people who don't cook that's the hardest thing about Paleo, but I cook so it's just as easy for me to cook Paleo than what I used to cook. Sometimes when I've been off Paleo or haven't worked out in a week or two it's hard to get back on, but I remind myself that I just really like how it feels to move my body. I like that empowered felling. I just really like that now.

Dali: Awesome. I think once you're used to working out, you know, the beginning of something is always the hardest part, but once you're used to it, and you're aware of how good it makes you feel, you want to feel that way more often. So, the consistency and the good feeling association with the activity or diet definitely helps you to continue being more consistent.

Melanie: Yeah, and on the diet, if I am even tempted with something, I always ask myself, is this going to be worth how I know I'm going to feel after I eat it? And, quite honestly, sometimes the answer is yes. But more often it's no. It's not going to be worth how I'm going to feel. It's not going to be worth the headache. It's not going to be worth the aching joints.

Dali: So, overall, Melanie, how do you think your journey has changed you as either a mom, wife, business owner or just as Melanie?

Melanie: Well, it's reinforced that when I set my mind to doing something, I can do it. Whether that's finishing the workout that I am certain is going to kill me or giving up foods that I really didn't think I could live without. So, it's that, like I said, I'm very empowered. And it has shown me that I am way stronger than I thought I was.

And it has allowed me to be a role model. It's allowed me to be a role model, especially, for my daughter. I am an amazing and very strong new woman.

Dali: Absolutely. You're showing her so much, and she's looking up to you. So, you're passing along that healthier lifestyle. Yes, awesome!

Any advice you would give someone who was in your shoes, or is in your shoes, when you were just starting your journey? Anything to help motivate her or get her going? What would you tell that person?

Melanie: I would say the most important part of any change is deciding. Just make a decision and then align your energy with it. And once you decide, find people to support you. The owner at the gym, she's been instrumental. And then there have been other great coaches who don't let me quit. They stay with me at the end of the workout. And the community there is great.

And Dali, I just need to tell you this story. Find a great community to work out in, or work with, because I remember the first time – this is like my first couple months – we were doing overhead squats in the workout, and it was one of those workouts where everyone was done, the next class was waiting, and I'm doing these overhead squats. It's my first time doing this exercise, and at the end, I remember I did my last squat, and I dropped the bar. Everyone, the people waiting for the class and the people that had been in my class working out with me, every single person there applauded.

And I was like, "Where else?" I mean like there is nowhere I'd get this support from. As a mom, there is nowhere else in my life I get that. My daughter doesn't applaud when I put dinner on the table!

So, make the decision and align your energy with it. Also, find a supportive community of people who are just going to cheer for you, and who will motivate you when you're feeling frustrated, or weak or whatever.

And there are days I go in, and when I go back, I know I'm going to have to say to my trainer, "look, I just want an 'ease-in' workout." I'm always clear about what I need and always listen to my body and advocate for myself. We're doing a workout the other day, and she's like we're going to do this, and I'm like "no ma'am. No, we're not. How? Because that's not going to happen."

Yeah, that is what I would say. Make the decision and align your energy, find your supportive community and someone who's going to cheer for you, but also support you when you're feeling frustrated. And listen to your internal wisdom.

I thought you'd get a kick out of this story being a trainer, Dali. Someone saying, "yup, no, that's not happening. Yep."

Dali: (Laughter). Love it. Thank you so much, Melanie, for sharing your story and advice.

By Dali Burgado, CPT

Interview with Rachel Brown

Rachel is a 40-year-old mother of 4, wife, and Health and Wellness Coach

Rachel defeated busyness and past failures. Rachel lost 25 lbs.

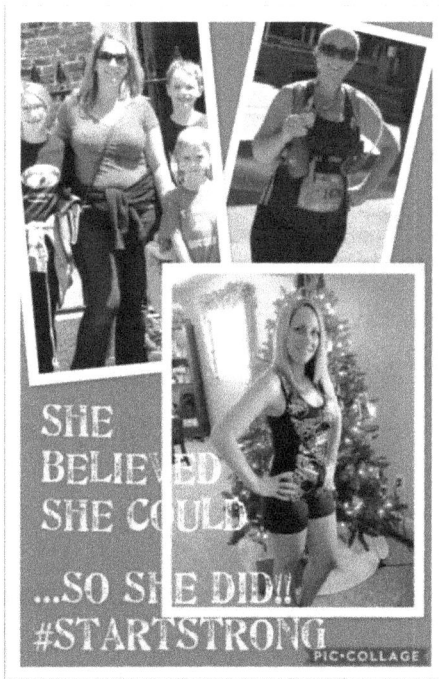

BEFORE & AFTER

Dali: Today, I have with me Rachel Brown. Rachel is a friend of mine, and we recently reconnected on Facebook.

So, Rachel is a fellow nutrition coach. She started her weight loss journey last year, and has made super huge strides. I wanted to reach out to Rachel because as soon as I had reconnected with her I saw the cool things that she was doing, and I'm like "Oh, wow, how crazy it is that we're both like on this big health kick." So, I want to share her story with you.

Dali: Rachel, what motivated you to begin your journey?

Rachel: Well, what really motivated me is I had, of course like a lot of women, after having children started the battle of wanting to lose weight and regain some of that youth and whatnot. And I had lost a bunch of weight a few years ago, and it was hard to do it. It took me a long time to lose weight the first time, and I was at home at the time. I prepped, and chopped, and did everything I was supposed to do. I worked out five days a week, and so it was really hard for me. And I lost a whole bunch of weight.

And it felt really good. I just swore I would never gain it back because of how hard it was. But then what happened was life took over—a move and inconvenient living, and I ended up just eating out all the time. So, I put all the weight back on. And it turns out at the beginning of the summer, I had gained all the weight back that I had lost plus 10 pounds.

So, I was at my max weight, and I just did not want to be there anymore. I could just feel myself not feeling well—my body starts to hurt at a certain weight. I can really start to feel the pressure on my knees when I'm heavier, so I really knew I had to make a change. So, that's what motivated me to get started was I did not want to go up another pants size. That was kind of the big thing. I did not want to gain another pound. So, that's really where the turning point was and what kicked me into gear at that point in time.

Dali: Was it during a particular season? Sometimes certain things going on in your life can push you there.

Rachel: Well, I had switched into a full-time job from a part-time job probably about three to four months prior to that. I was starting to get busier, and I was trying to figure out a way to make exercising and eating healthy work into my new busy life. So, it was at the beginning of summer, we had just gotten back from a big vacation, and an opportunity came for me to train for a race, and that's when I decided to kick it into high gear and start.

Dali: Cool. That goal that you had for the race, I bet that pushed you even further, right, because you had a specific goal in mind?

Rachel: Yeah, you know, I never ran a race before, and so I wanted to try something new. Some friends of mine were doing this half-marathon, and it was kind of an "everybody was going to be walking it event," but I didn't want to do that because that would take too long. So, I decided to start training so I could run it, and I just put my blinders on. At that particular time, I didn't want to implement too many healthy things into my life because I was time-deprived. I still was really busy working a full-time job. It was still really challenging to eat a lot of healthier foods.

I was eating less, and I cut out junk. To me, exercising and eating right always goes hand-in-hand, and I can't do one without the other. So, I can't eat like a pig and exercise, right. I just can't. It's the weirdest thing. I can't go exercise while I'm pigging out and vice versa.

So, at that point in time, I was kind of mixing up smoothies in the morning with Greek Yogurt and some fruit and stuff like that and then at lunch I would do a salad. At work, I would hit the salad bar and put a bunch of chicken in my salad, and then I would have whatever for dinner. But because I was working out four days a week training for this run for about an hour to an hour and a half four times a week, the weight just started to come off. The first 20 pounds just started to come off at that point in time. And that was June to the race was the first weekend of September.

Dali: So, looking back to when you first got started, do you remember feeling a particular way about your current fitness level and anything that really encouraged you to get moving?

Rachel: I can specifically remember how painful it was. Because I had had so much weight on my body, and I remember running and I was just like gosh, if I can just lose 10 pounds I will feel so much better. I always equated that extra 10 pounds to a 10-pound bag of potatoes. So, I was always like that's pretty heavy. And I was like if I could just lose that, I'll feel better.

And I can also remember just feeling overwhelmed with how much I wanted to lose weight because it's really hard to stay motivated when you think about how much weight you have to lose. And so, I would do things like reward myself for the small milestones. So, every time I lost 10 pounds, I would go buy myself a new fitness t-shirt.

Dali: Awesome.

Rachel: You know it was just kind of a good – like I love cute fitness clothes, so I would just go buy a shirt because shirts were one of those things. The good news about fitness clothes, and some shirts, is they're kind of forgiving, so you can wear them a little bigger or they stretch. So, I can wear them for a long time. Yeah, so that was kind of what I used to stay motivated. I focused on small milestones and rewarded myself each time I met a new milestone.

Dali: Yeah, so feeling like as you run, and you know running is taxing for anybody, but when you run and you know that there's weight that you want to lose and you'll feel better having lost that weight, it gets a little tough if you're at a place where you feel like you really need to lose that weight. It makes it harder to run.

Rachel: And I can remember telling my dad—my dad's an ultra-runner—I can remember telling him. I was just like it's not my lung capacity. That actually caught up quickly. I felt good from the waist up, but I just remember my legs hurting because of the weight. So, I would just kind of imagine -- I mean I would do it a lot where I'd be running and I would just imagine what it would be like losing the weight. Or I joked with some friends picturing the fat falling off me as I'm running. So, just different things like that helped me stay motivated.

Dali: That's a wonderful visual. I love it! Yes.

Rachel: And so, I just would think of those things. As you're running, you just kind of think about those things. And then each week that goes by and the mileage that builds or the pounds that come off, it just gets more and more encouraging to keep going. So, that's just how that went.

Dali: So, at that time do you remember having any fears at all?

Rachel: Yeah, I would say probably one of the biggest fears I had at that time was just that it would be like any other attempt over the previous three, four years to lose weight that I would get going for only a week or two and then just stop or that nothing would happen. I feared that I would never get the weight off, and I could remember feeling that way during that time. But each week I also knew I had committed to a race. There's nothing like putting money out there to motivate you!

And so I had committed to that. So, it was just each week, I just wanted to keep going and going. So, I just kept going. That's what I always tell everybody. Just keep going. Like Finding Dory.

Dali: Funny! Were there any other fears that you can remember, and how did you overcome maybe that nagging voice in your head? I know it pops up often.

Rachel: For me, the fear set in a little later. So, it wasn't so much at the beginning but maybe when I was at my halfway point.

I'm a pretty confident person, so that keeps me going, but when I got closer to the fall where I was getting ready to transition into an extremely busy time. At that point in my life, the fear crept in. Being a mom of four, having full-time work, and preparing to start school again part-time was stressful. And I hadn't been to college in 20 years. So, I was getting ready to do that, and it was scary.

I was worried at that point, and that's when I was kind of like, "Crap, the race is going to be over, and I'm not really eating my best now," and I started looking for solutions at that point in time for my health because I knew that my fitness level was going to decrease after the race. It was right when fall was starting, and I was going from training mode to work and school mode. There were some days where I would leave for work at 8:00 am in the morning, and I wouldn't get home until 10:00 pm at night because of school. So, I really needed to have a solution that was easy for me to help with the diet part of it or my healthy eating. So, that's when I started worrying at that point in time. But, I just looked for a solution to continue my health journey.

Dali: So, between the busyness of the life, the fall, work, and being done with the race some fears crept in, but you found something to help you stay the course and reach the next goal? It makes sense that when you're super busy the diet isn't going to be all that great. So those were a few of your obstacles?

Rachel: Right. Yeah, and that was probably the biggest obstacle I had was at that point in time. During the summer, I had a lot more time, and there were more daylight hours. I had more time to work out, especially running when outside and that's when you need to do those long runs. But come fall, everything was going to change.

So, I started a new chapter in the fall and began incorporating nutritional supplements. At that point in time, I started to get really excited even though it was challenging because at that point I couldn't get to the gym as much. But because I could find a solution, I stayed on track, I continued to see my weight go down, and I felt like for the first time ever I was going to meet a health goal. Before that, I'd never set a real goal I just usually set out to lose weight.

Rachel: The last time I had done that was when I was a stay-at-home mom. I went to the gym for an hour and a half to two hours every morning. I pulled out all the ingredients out of the fridge to make nice, healthy, well-rounded meals, and I wrote down every single calorie that I ate. I mean, I had a journal and everything. And I did that for months. And at that point in time, I just knew, my life could not sustain that this time. So, I was worried. How was I going to make this happen?

And so, enter my nutritional supplements, and that just really happened to help me find an easy solution to help me continue. And not only that, but get even more nutrients than I would have ever had with any other meal like making a salad or something like that. So, it really helped me and, more importantly, it also helped me do it with my husband. That was something we always struggled with was getting on the same page with our health.

Either he was on a health kick or I was, and most of the time it was me. So, most of the time I was the one who was trying to lose 10 pounds or something. So, it was really great that I found something that we could do together, and I spent a lot of time researching it because I knew I'd need to convince him. So, I sat down with him, and I said "Okay look, I want to do this. I think we should do this together," and he was open to it. And he's done amazing. He's lost 39 pounds.

But for me, I finally at Christmas time I hit a health goal, and I hit it in the time frame I wanted to hit it. And that had never really happened. It had always been like I'm going to lose 10 pounds in 30 days and I would lose six. And I think the difference this time was that I was realistic in my weight loss.

I didn't do anything crazy where I was trying to say I was going to lose five pounds a week or anything like that. I mean I really lost about one and a half to two pounds a week. It wasn't anything outrageous, but that's hard to sustain for people because they want instant gratification. So, for me, and I'd say most people, I was just talking about this the other day, with summer coming, this is when people should be thinking about getting healthy if they want to be summer-ready. But what most people do is we're like 30 days out from a vacation, we're like, "Oh my God, I've got to lose 30 pounds!"

And I ask, "Well how long did it take you to put that on?!" And I still struggle, I'm still learning how to eat healthy and how to eat that extra meal that's healthy.

I still love junk food, so it's hard sometimes to get past that.

Dali: So, you had some obstacles, but you could overcome them, and I know you mentioned the importance of supplements, but how was it that you changed from the way you were eating to the way you are eating now?

Rachel: What changed with my eating was eating smaller meals. And that was a big part of it because instead of going back for seconds or thirds, because my supplements filled me up, it provided the nutrients for me. Typically, when we're hungry we want nutrients, not empty calories. And because it provided me with nutrients, when it came time for dinner—and late-night snacking is a downfall of mine—it satisfied me so I wouldn't have the late-night snack.

I would have my dinner, and I would eat whatever the family was eating. I just wouldn't have seconds, and I wouldn't have thirds. And then I also wouldn't have late night snacks or eat candy. During this time leading up to Christmas, I had my anniversary, I had my birthday, my son's birthday, Halloween, Thanksgiving, Christmas, my daughter's birthday, and New Year's all wrapped in there, and I still managed to lose the weight because I would have those meals, but I wouldn't forego everything I was working on.

I'd go out and have a nice dinner for my birthday or anniversary and probably eat a little too much and feel full, but I would get back on it the next day. I wouldn't just be like,

"Oh well, the weekend's shot. I'll just eat bad tomorrow too." I just stayed incredibly focused during that time.

Dali: So, you had good self-control. You would have your cheat meals, and you would take advantage of those holidays, but it seems you are focused.

Rachel: Yeah, I can be. I can be focused, especially if I've got a goal in mind or something like that, and about halfway through, it really transitioned to me desiring to share with other people because of the community I was in. Which, I think is also key. You need to be surrounded by people who are like-minded. It's hard to hang out with people that are—and it doesn't mean you can't hang out with them—but it's really hard to hang out with those people that like to eat a lot, and go out to eat and that kind of thing.

When you're trying to eat healthy, that can be a big issue. For us, that was a lot of the issue. Leading up until the beginning of that year, we were living with family and there was a lot of well, "We'll just get take out tonight." So, there was a lot of unhealthy eating because of our environment. And so being around this healthy community I've gotten to know, these friends that are striving to be healthier, striving to lose weight, build muscle, just age well, whatever it is, has helped.

All those things, just being around these awesome, like-minded people who talk about health all the time just really helped to keep me accountable. And plus, I wanted to set a good example for those I was coaching, so that also helps to keep me accountable too.

Dali: Absolutely. Cool. Now, if you were to think about your journey, how did you change as a woman, as a wife?

Rachel: Hm. Yeah, it was funny, when I was reviewing these questions actually, for this particular one it was like, "Uh, I don't know how to answer that. I was like, I don't know." It's a deep question.

Dali: Did you feel like you became a little more focused or was there something that you conquered or something inside you that you didn't know you had? How did this whole journey change who you are?

Rachel: Yeah. Well, a couple of things changed. Okay, so one, I'll be 40 later this year, so one of the things -- and actually we were at a chiropractic appointment tonight and it happened to be kind of like a presentation about just what chiropractic is and what it means. And I'd always thought it was a little bit hokey to go to a chiropractor. But, it just really got me thinking about just our overall health. So, one thing that's really changed about me is just health in general or how I view health. I'm more open to learning about health, overall.

Before, it was always just about a number, and even when I talk to people I can see it in them when I'm talking to people who I'm introducing this healthy lifestyle to, I can see it in them. It's just about losing weight, it's about getting into those jeans that you wore a few years ago, and it starts small. And that's what it was for me. I just wanted to be thin again. It started small.

But as you go on, now it's more about just being healthy because I'm getting older. I don't want a lot of those same struggles. I don't want diabetes, I don't want high blood pressure for my husband because he really struggles with that and heart problems. That's what it's more about for me now. So, I'm thinking about things more in an overall health-conscious way and even for my family and for others too. So that's really what has changed with me is that I'm really looking at the world through health now versus just the outside image. More of the inside and learning a lot about that, your inside health.

Dali: So, if you can look back, what kept you motivated in your journey?

Rachel: Well, initially it was wanting to be able to run the race. And that's what kept me focused. After, as I went on, and especially once I transitioned how I was eating and what I was eating, it was other people. I mean, it's the community I'm part of. And that was really what kept me going. Also, it was my husband and really wanting to do this with him and not fall off and let him fall off, because what usually happens in relationships is that if you fall off, they fall off too. So, if I decide if I don't want to do this anymore, it's only a matter of time. He was very determined and very disciplined, so I wanted to keep that up for him. Plus, I started to see that other people I was meeting really respond to this kind of thing on social media, and even before I was trying to build a business or anything like that, I could see that people are really interested in their health, so it motivated me and kept me going. I was encouraging other people.

Dali: Absolutely.

Rachel: You know, that was a big part of it. I'm very honest about how, "Okay, yeah. I didn't do very well this week, but let's keep going." And I'm very honest about that and just being real with other people that I'm coaching or even just not coaching, just other people in general. I can see it sometimes. Even if I'm not personally working with them, suddenly, it's like I've reached out to them to talk to them, and now I see them posting things about changing their diet or they're taking steps or whatever it is. And it's not that I'm necessarily influencing them --but maybe I am, maybe I'm not. But, it's nice to see people really trying to do something healthy.

Dali: Absolutely. I think it's rewarding, right.

Rachel: Yeah. Someone recently told me I have a tremendous amount of grit, and I think that's a lot of it too. I just make my mind up about something, and I dig in and do it. And it's been incredibly exciting to lose weight and regain some of that and feeling like, "I've got this." I'm not going to go back to the way it was now. So, it's a really good feeling.

Dali: Awesome. Now, I know you didn't have a coach for your running. I know you mentioned you use an app. And if you want to share a little bit about that, I'd like to hear it. But I do want to know, do you have any other coaches or mentors that help keep you motivated on your journey?

Rachel: Yes. I have a team, and we have people that I reach out to, and they've been able to help me like if I've got questions about what I'm supposed to do or if I need a little motivation for certain things. I have some people who help encourage me. It was just more of the community that kept me motivated. Whether it's being on the Facebook page and you know there's someone who says they're being impacted by your posts. Like the other day, I posted a picture of my challenge before and after pictures, which show a little more of my body than I've posted on public social media. And I remember when I posted that in our private group page, and my coworker who's in that group—I have some people that are in it that are just checking things out—and my coworker said, "I thought you said you would never post that kind of picture," and it was like, "I know. I did. I said I never would."

And then because of that though, my girlfriend came to me and she was like, "I can't believe you shared that. That was so inspiring. I want to do this with you." And she's lost 13 pounds, and she loves it and she's feeling great. And so that's what it is really, just the community of people has really been life-changing to me as well as being a part of that and seeing my husband change. And now he's concerned about his health and stepping out, and we're talking about health with the chiropractor and our whole family now. We're going to seminars and really checking these things out because it's just becoming a whole family thing. They're my coaches.

Dali: Awesome. Well, what final pieces of advice would you give someone who has just started on their journey and maybe isn't super focused? I think you and I are a lot alike in the fact that we're focused, determined, and then set that goal and get it done. And we're both coaches. What would you recommend to someone who just needs that little extra motivation starting out?

Rachel: You know, I would say what I've shared with people who are just getting started in their journey, and I've known a couple people that are just really having a hard time getting going now. What I would do is just really keep your focus one day at a time and just really celebrate the little wins. It's hard to do, especially if you've got a big goal. It's hard to be excited about one pound. It's hard to be excited about two and, "Oh, I only lost two pounds this week when really at this point I should be losing five! Because it's the beginning of my weight loss journey!" That's what I'd say—just really take things one day at a time.

The other thing that I tell people all the time is just keep going. Keep going. And because that's where you'll get it is if you keep going. Don't give up. And we do this too many times, and I've been there. That's why I know this. Too many times after 30 days or a few weeks it's kind of like, "this is too hard, I don't want to do this anymore!" And people just quit. Or, "I've had a bad week." I hear that a lot too. "Oh, I had such a bad week, I got all off track." And I'm like, "You know what? Don't wait until Monday. Diets, contrary to popular belief, can start on other days of the week besides Monday! Just start tomorrow. It's okay."

And I'm always just very encouraging to that. That's what I would say and that's how I would be. It's okay. You know what, I actually had half a pizza to myself last night because I do. I have those nights where I just ate way too much. This is what I always tell everybody is just keep going. Keep at it. Don't give up. Find something that works for you and stick to it. Everyone needs a routine. You need a plan. But just find it, stick to it, and just keep going. That's what I would say.

Dali: So, one day at a time, celebrate the small wins, and keep going. Awesome. I appreciate you taking time out of your busy day to get interviewed and sharing your story for the book.

Interview with Tina Walker

A mid-40s working woman, motivator, and caregiver.

Tina defeated depression and negativity. Tina lost 24 lbs., recently completed her first 5K race, and is currently working on losing the next 30 lbs.

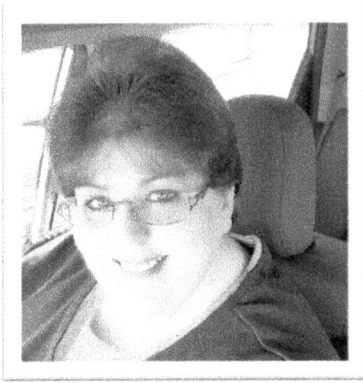

BEFORE

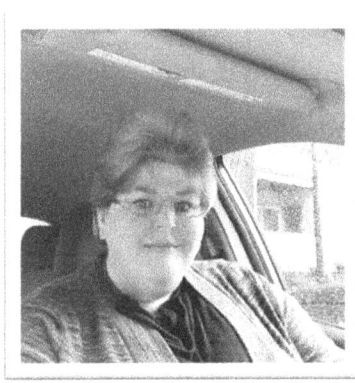

AFTER

Dali: Hey, this is Dali Burgado here with Dali Burgado Fitness. Today I have, Tina Walker, and Tina is a friend and client of mine, so I'm really excited for this interview because, ever since day one, Tina has been excited—you know, of course everyone has their ups and downs—but Tina is super motivational and she even created her own Facebook group to help her in her fitness journey and help inspire others in their journey as well. She has her own hash tag #TeamTina. Tina has lost 24 pounds in the last 12 weeks and is working on losing her next 30! I just wanted to welcome Tina ask her a few questions.

Dali: Tina, what motivated you to begin your fitness journey?

Tina: Well basically, what motivated me in my journey is looking at my life and wanting more. I put my life on hold for others as a caregiver, and that made my health go down. It's a journey to get back up to where I used to be. I've always been overweight, but just to have a different perspective in life and how to go about fulfilling my dreams and my purpose here in life.

Dali: What feelings do you remember having right before you started your fitness journey that were encouraging you in the beginning?

Tina: In the beginning, I felt I had started my fitness journey somewhat blind-sighted by my previous fitness failures and the fear of not being able to accomplish anything. But my faith through Christ is what basically gave me, and gives me, the motivation to push through every day.

Dali: Did you have any other fears in the beginning, and if so, what were they?

Tina: My fears were not so much about my health problems because I really don't have any other issues other than arthritis. My fears were around the injuries that I previously experienced as a child with broken bones and the emotional weight that I had carried. I would wonder if I would be able to perform enough exercises to actually keep up with this fitness journey and go over and beyond my expectations to succeed. Would I even succeed?

Dali: How did you overcome that doubt and fear as you went through the journey?

Tina: I decided to put the fears on the backburner and let my positive overtake the fears in saying that I can't do something. I'd tell myself that *I can do it*! You know, just having that whole, complete mindset reverse that I am forgiving of myself for the things that happened to me in my past. I would tell myself that I'm an overcomer, and I will succeed just by having that accountability with myself and with others through fellowship.

Dali: You mentioned a strong word, "overcomer." I know sometimes it's hard for a lot of people to overpower the fears or overpower the negative thoughts that they're having with good ones that will serve them. Do you have any tips for someone who, maybe negativity is all they know, and it's hard for them to stop being afraid or start doing something they know they should? Do you have any tips on getting to that state where you say, "You know what, I *am* an overcomer! I'm pushing my fears aside!"?

Tina: My tip is you basically – well – I looked at my life as the trauma I faced as a child, and I said that if I allowed that to keep going on in my life, if I continued dwelling on that negativity, that whatever happens in my life, I'm letting them hold me hostage in my ability to move forward. So, look to the brighter things that keep you motivated. You need to seek freedom and break the chains of bondage. You need to let go and be free because the past and your negative feelings are bondage that are holding you back in fulfilling your purpose and even having the willpower for having a better and healthier outlook on life.

Dali: That's super powerful, Tina. Looking at the beginning of your journey, you overcoming your fears, and being super positive, what kind of obstacles did you come across? Because we all come across these obstacles, in the beginning, especially.

Tina: I think the biggest obstacle for me was the gym. Having that mindset of, "Oh, I'm being judged by others," but your worst critic is yourself. You're judging yourself. You know, you're not going in there to prove something to them. You're going in there to prove something to yourself, and that you can do this and you're in charge of your life. Granted, God gave you that life, but you're in charge of your life and how you live your life.

Dali: Absolutely. So, getting the courage to get to the gym was an obstacle. Was there anything else that, you know, you talk about others judging you and overcoming that, was there anything else that you feel set you back at any point and you had to overcome? A small hurdle?

Tina: Well my small hurdle was really changing also the eating aspects of this health journey because there were times when the depression would kick in, and I wouldn't eat or I would over eat because I was emotional and just eating the wrong stuff. So now I have the mindset, and I have the willpower to make better changes and choices in what I'm eating and drinking. I went through a complete transformation of my mind and what had to be done to succeed, to be efficient in my ability, in my health, and in my wellness.

Dali: So, I know that comes up a lot. It takes effort to change your eating habits and getting used to eating different foods. What helped you get more of the nutritious food in your diet?

Tina: Time, preparation, and really looking at the ingredients of meal planning and a time frame because working retail, you have hours and times where you're so busy you don't have time to prepare. And it's just making yourself accountable to doing the meal planning and setting it out instead of just going out and picking up fast food or going to a restaurant.

Dali: So, setting aside that time to prepare helped you incorporate the foods better throughout the weeks?

Tina: Yes. For sure.

Dali: Ok, so, Tina, who did you become in this process? Because I know you have the Team Tina group, and I see everything that you post on Facebook because I'm in the group. And we talk about the journey because life is a journey, right? Everything is a journey. You don't get instant results. It's a process. You go to the gym, you eat healthier, you work on your mindset, on those beliefs and shoving those negative beliefs and those fears and getting past that.

You motivate a lot of people through your posts, and you're reaching other people, so how is it that you stay motivated throughout the journey despite the obstacles? Despite the fears?

Tina: I stay motivated through prayer, for sure. And through devotionals. To me, that gives me the power to go over and beyond my own expectations because I have the strength through Christ who strengthens me. It's just, I can't do enough throughout the day to really glorify myself but glorifying him. It's a weird but not a weird sensation that you get whenever you've accomplished something that you've had set in your mind for 20-30 years down the road that you're physically, mentally and spiritually ready to start doing something and start living a healthy lifestyle.

Dali: That's one of my favorite Bible Verses. I hear and see your posts a lot, and I see how you live every day, but for people who are either reading the book or hearing this, do you want to share a little bit on your faith journey and how that's helped you become a stronger woman in your fitness journey?

Tina: Yeah, I can go a little bit into it. As a child, I was physically and mentally abused by my mother, and I had some trauma as a child that basically put me on a spiral to where I didn't feel that I was good enough, and so I chose food over anything. That was my comfort, and it took me 41 years to start living and break free from that and start living the life that I wanted and I know that I deserve through Christ because I'm a God daughter.

By Dali Burgado, CPT

It's just when my husband passed away in 2010, I had taken care of him. I put my life completely on hold because I felt that's what God wanted me to do, and basically when he passed away I turned away from Christ because I was so upset with God that I did everything that he needed me to do. And I also had a miscarriage in that marriage. So, it took me two and a half years after or a year and a half after my husband passed away, that on my birthday I went to church and I accepted Christ back into my life, which He never left me.

From that day forward, I said, and my quote was, when getting re-baptized, "I am seeing my life now through Christ as he gave me life on November 13th." Without Him, he was my joy, because I accepted Christ when I was five-years-old, and things started happening at the age of seven, and it went until I was maybe 10. So, having that faith journey up and down as a child and then totally disregarding my faith when I got older, it's almost like I've been reborn as a child through my faith, and building me back up to where I'm more positive now in my faith journey. And He's my go-to whenever I'm defeated or anything. I just give it all to him.

Dali: Yes! Definitely. I'm so glad that you shared that with us. I just kind of felt called to ask that question because you're so strong in your faith, and I know, for me too, it's a huge part of my life, and something that I lean on when I'm in the dumps and kind of lean on my own strength, which you know, we talk about fitness and getting strong and everything, but if you're not strong spiritually, then what good is it? I believe that very strongly and you exhibit that every day, and you may not see it, but you are encouraging and inspiring so many other people not only in their fitness journey, but also in their spiritual journey as well.

Tina: Right. (With a smile).

Dali: And that's really cool! So, you overcame those obstacles, you leaned heavily on your faith and your positive mindset. Your faith is what keeps you going. How has the last 12 weeks transformed you at all, as a woman, either as a woman of faith or just Tina? How has this transformed Tina?

Tina: Well, it's basically transformed me into having better control of my life. Making that time for myself in the morning, making that time in preparing my food, making that time and commitment to go to the gym. I just have a better mindset. I have a better goal in life because of the Bible verse that I use and I put on my group. It's Proverbs 3:8 – "This will bring health to your body and nourishment to your bones." Regardless of that verse itself, it may be talking about health and fitness, but that's also talking about your inner spirit, too.

Because you're rebuilding the outside but you're also rebuilding the inside too.

Dali: Super powerful. I'm going to ask you this, but I know you know the answer, and I know the answer. Did you have a coach? And what role did your coach play?

Tina: The role that my coach played was a big part of who I am today because she made me really sit down and focus on what I want, how I want to do it, and when I want to do it. It's that accountability that, you know, that interaction that she has with me in the gym, outside of the gym. She's just an overall joy in my life. Granted there are times when we do some exercises, and I'm not really enjoying it. I enjoy the push that she gives me because that's God pushing her to push me!

Dali: Thank you, Tina. I'm so proud of you! For those of you hearing or reading, Tina's coach is the person interviewing her right now. I appreciate you, and I was so looking forward to this interview with you because I knew we were going to talk about some deeper things and faith and how important that is to you and me, and I'm excited to have this one in the book. This is the last interview, and it's the most special one to me, at least.

Tina: Thank you.

Dali: Any other parting advice that you would give someone who has been wanting to make changes in their health and maybe they're just hung up on something and haven't made that commitment? What would you tell that person?

Tina: I would tell them, basically do what I did. Look at yourself in the mirror and ask those hard questions or those questions that you want to improve upon. You're your own accountability partner. Make that commitment to yourself that you want to change because if you don't accept the challenge for yourself personally, you may not see the change you want to see.

And if your goal is to lose weight, have a visual for your weight loss because the scale is an over-weight person's biggest demon -- is basically what I call it. For instance, put marbles in a jar each time you lose a pound or an inch somewhere. And each time you lose weight -- use that, don't use the scale as what you've gained or what you've lost. Go by staying positive for the weight you have lost, and don't focus on the negative.

Dali: Absolutely! That's the reason you don't focus on the negative, and I like that you mentioned the visual. And you have that very creative way to motivate. You found that on Pinterest or something, right? I love the glass jar with the marbles in it to symbolize the weight that you keep losing. And then you can see that. But even in your progress pictures, you can see the differences throughout your journey, as you exercise more and continue to eat healthier you're transforming. Of course, you're not always going to eat 100% healthy. We're all allowed a splurge. But the important thing is if you strive for it, you continue to work on it, and work on yourself, and you keep at it. So, that's good. Anything else that maybe is on your mind that God's put on your heart? A quote?

Tina: I have one quote that I want to share it is, "The first step in having courage is to make the changes with the strength to see your goal through and keeping your faith alive. It will all turn out for the best."

Chapter 11: How They Defeated It and So Will You!

"You see, you can at times experience a moment
of regression because you are human. But as
long as you recognize that defeat is only
temporary, reverse the negative experience, and
you get back on track, you've won!"

—Dali Burgado, Author, Certified Personal
Trainer, Certified Weight Management
Specialist, and Mentor

Each of these women experienced common fears and challenges. They were motivated by similar things while each having different inspiration as they went through their fitness journey. Collectively, however, at the end of each stage was positive and permanent change. Each of these ladies gave you advice. I want to take this time to summarize some of those common fears and challenges, as well as motivations, to help you defeat whatever it is you are trying to defeat as you embark on your fitness journey. You are not alone.

For most of these women, their defining moment when they said enough was enough, was for the most part, the physical pain due to weight gain. And at some point, they felt the exhaustion and low energy that comes with being overweight. And for Ronnie, Rachel, and even myself, there was not only some physical but emotional weight and pain due to that weight gain too.

With Melanie, her defining moment was seeing how ill her mother got and not wanting to repeat that story herself. She also had achy joints. For Tina, she put herself second for far too long at her very own detriment. I know when I was pregnant and was at my heaviest, not too long ago, it was doctor's orders, and realizing I had lost the self-control and the discipline that I had gained throughout the last 5 years.

You see, you can at times experience a moment of regression because you are human. But as long as you recognize that defeat is only temporary, reverse the negative experience, and you get back on track, you've won! Reflecting on my two-month lapse in positivity early on in my last pregnancy, I realize it was only "momentary." If you compare that temporary defeat with the five years I've been on my fitness journey, the two months is a drop in the bucket. While I sat in my depression for two months, I got back up. I realized I needed to get past and defeat my fear. I also realized I wanted something bigger than me. I wanted to be a role model to other women in my family, and I wanted to get my pre-pregnancy body back. This is what motivated me to stick to what I already set for myself after my car accident but got a little side tracked by the temporary defeat.

Of course, there are going to be fears and challenges as you embark on any journey, not just fitness, but in life. And some of those common fears, when it comes to getting healthier, and you might already be concerned with, are:

- Will I find balance and consistency?
- How can I change the diet?
- What if I hit a plateau?
- What if I fail and I don't stick with this "fitness kick"?

All of us five ladies felt these fears at one point or another. And chances are you will too. But it's about how you get past these fears and start making progress. How do we stop focusing on the enormous goal and start focusing on the milestones? I hope that the first half of this book and the written exercises helped you find strategies to start thinking of ways to overcome those fears and challenges. I also hope you also found the interviews helpful and that they inspired you to find solutions.

Ronnie overcame her fear of not finding balance by planning. She actively planned her workouts around her family and lifestyle and found creative ways to exercise with her children and not allowing excuses to derail her. Melanie found a group challenge to motivate her to get over her fear of dieting. Rachel, found reward in visualizing the fat falling off as she ran every mile. Tina overcame being self-conscious by telling herself that her opinion mattered most, and she was really judging herself.

And each of these women found motivation in their families and the fact that they are role models to their children and community. In fact, each of these women advocate for being in a positive community to help motivate themselves. For Tina and myself, it is not only a community of friends and like-minded individuals, but also a community of faith, prayer and knowing that you are an overcomer no matter what obstacles you might face in life and in fitness.

What inspiration can you draw from these stories of each of these unique women?

_____

_____

_____

_____

_____

_____

_____

As these women experienced their journeys, they found inspiration in rewarding themselves for a job well done and for the reaching the small milestones. They all had the feeling that if I can do that; if I can do this, I can do anything! You see, once you see that you can really do something, it makes you want to do it more often and then try more challenging things.

For myself, inspiration comes through progress, taking pictures, and monitoring stats, measurements, and sharing my journey to inspire others. All the courageous ladies who were interviewed for this book were all inspired despite their obstacles, small hurdles, or fears.

> Once you start your journey, or you take
>
> your journey on supercharge, you realize
>
> how much stronger you are than you think
>
> you are.

And each of these women despite all the obstacles, small hurdles, and fears learned more about their true capabilities and about themselves. They all became more confident. Ronnie and Melanie became comfortable in their body. Ronnie learned to accept herself no matter what bullies used to tell her when she was young, and she regained balance in her busy life.

Once you start your journey, or you take your journey on supercharge, you realize how much stronger you are than you think you are. For Rachel, health became a lifestyle. She's learning more and more about health every day and sharing it with others. For Tina, her journey meant better control over her life. For myself, I gained that superwoman energy, the strength, and greater post-pregnancy self-confidence I once feared I wouldn't have. Due to this outlet of strength, I am still a personal trainer even though I went through a third pregnancy going on my 40s.

To leave you with some parting advice, here are some additional things and reminders to help you as you defeat whatever it is that you are trying to defeat. For one, let go of emotional weight as you let go of the physical weight. Ronnie let go of a lot of the insecurity and lack of confidence that she held baggage as a kid. The more fit and confident she became, the more baggage she dropped.

Remember to listen to your body and don't compare yourself to anyone else. Someone's day 1000 is not going to be your day one. Remember, it's all a decision, a conscious decision to drop the baggage, let go of fears, look for solutions, and get it done.

> Remember, it's all a decision, a conscious
>
> decision to drop the baggage, let go of
>
> fears, look for solutions, and get it done.

Accountability is huge, whether it's with a spouse like Rachel or with a friend, a group of friends or a fitness coach. Going through the journey with others and a community will help you become more accountable to yourself.

Being realistic with your weight loss goals is also important. Both Rachel and Tina realized this. When I'm coaching my girls, the goal is to lose the first 20 pounds and then work on celebrating the small accomplishments, whether its buying yourself little rewards, taking yourself to get a massage, or pedicures. Reward yourself for those milestones. Celebrate those small wins. As Rachel mentioned also, just keep going. Make a commitment to yourself. If you need to, hire a coach. Rely on your faith, and find a visual.

Sometimes it takes longer for us to really pick up steam and be at the point where we are all-in and all the pieces are aligned. Results come by much quicker if you have the motivation to go all-in like Melanie did with her eight-week diet challenge. But, what matters most is just starting.

The toughest part about a fitness journey or any journey, whether it's advancing your education or career, is starting. All the fears that are involved in something new will be there, and all the challenges you know that are going to be there will be there too, but instead, focus on what's possible. Focus on that strength and confidence you'll gain. Focus on the person you want to become, and see yourself as that person now. Focus on what you can do now! Anticipate how you will overcome expected challenges like I had you do on page 67.

Always look for solutions when you face a hurdle. Like Ronnie, as a teacher during summer time, she found activities where she could incorporate exercise with her kids. She found walking trails, parks, where she and her kids could work out together. So, she had no excuse to stop working out during the rough summers. Then she also set that example for her children, setting new traditions and habits that her children will learn for a lifetime.

Rachel found a supplement and diet that allowed her to keep weight off and continue to lose weight with a less active lifestyle after she went back to college while being a mom of 4 and working full time.

Always practice shifting your perspective so that you look away from the challenges and towards the solutions. This is an art and form of creativity that you will have once you're clear on your WHY. When you know how badly you want to achieve your goal and you align your focus and energy, your subconscious and conscious will work for you and arrive at creative solutions to those small hurdles. That is all they really are – small hurdles and not big challenges.

Remember, when you feel down or feel like you've come across a challenge, ask yourself, "What can I do now to work towards my goal of _____." It's perspective!

Look away from the fears and look towards that positive change that you will gain. You were born to succeed. The only thing left to do now is decide who it is you want to become. Now, go *Defeat It!*

With All My Heart, I Thank you! And My Gifts for You!

I truly hope you got a lot of this book. If you really found value in this book and workbook, please provide a 5-Star review on Amazon.com.

If this book helps you find your breakthrough, please email me your testimony at:

daliburgadofitness@daliburgado.com.

If you'd like me to feature your testimony on my site, please let me know!

When writing your testimony and review, consider what you learned, embraced, and what part of this book made the most impact on your life.

- Where were you before reading this book and what is your current perspective now?
- How did you feel while you read the book and worked on the workbook questions?
- How did reading this book change you moving forward?

If you're looking for additional help and guidance in your fitness journey, you may reach out and inquire about hiring me to help coach you along the way! I offer online, and on-on-one personal training and nutrition and meal planning services.

Find me on Facebook:

Personal Profile:

https://www.facebook.com/dali.burgado

Dali Burgado Fitness Fan Page:

https://www.facebook.com/DaliBurgadoFitness

Join the Defeat It! Facebook Community

Defeat It! Fan Page:

https://www.facebook.com/defeatitbook

Find my websites at:

http://www.daliburgado.com

http://www.defeatitbook.com

My Gifts to You:

1. Download your free workbook with all the questions and resources mentioned in this book here: https://defeatitbook.com/workbook

2. If you've completed your workbook and email it to me at daliburgadofitness@daliburgado.com, you can schedule a free 15 Minute Clarity Call with me (by appointment only). Just click on the blue "Contact" button on the bottom right of my site to schedule your appointment: http://www.daliburgado.com/

3. If you're ready to start or advance your journey with me, you can schedule a 30-minute transformation call with me the same way as noted above.

By Dali Burgado, CPT

About the Author – Dali Burgado, CPT

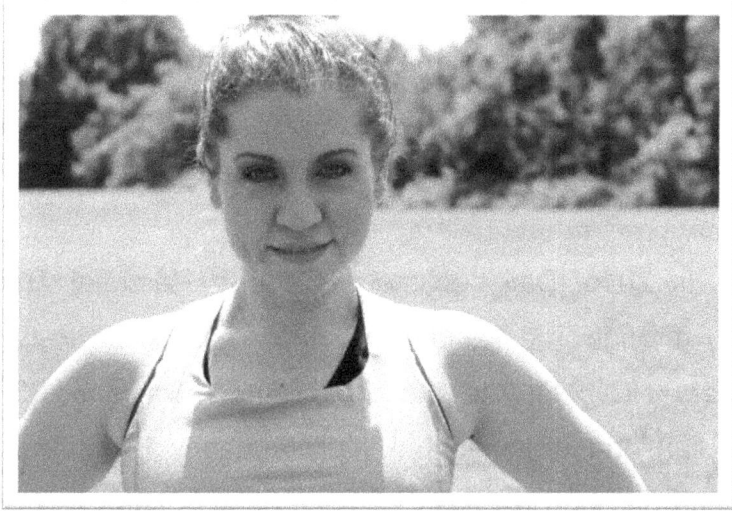

Dali Burgado is a mother of three children ages 12, 10, and 9 months, a foster mom of an 18-year-old, wife, and a perpetual student. She graduated from Colgate University in 2001 with a Bachelor of Arts. Even though she majored in Political Science and began her career as a Capitol Hill Assistant, she quickly learned Politics was not her forte.

From the 2000s into 2008 she worked different home-based businesses from home party sales to wholesale vacation sales and found she loved to learn all she could about marketing, sales, and psychology. She immersed herself into the online marketing space and landed several IT jobs based on her self-taught online marketing skills, which she had utilized for her own business ventures.

In 2005, she was married, had her first daughter, Christine, and in 2006 had Luis, her son. In 2016, she had her third child, Angel. After a near-death car accident, in 2012 Dali decided that she was blessed to survive and found a passion for God, fitness, and sharing her knowledge on health and fitness.

In 2015, Dali became a Certified Personal Trainer (CPT) through The National Council for Certified Personal Trainers (NCCPT). After the birth of Angel, Dali shed 33 lbs. (40 total) and regained her pre-pregnancy fit body back. Through diet and exercise 22 minutes at a time, 3 times a week, Dali became a role-model to her friends, family, and community. It was during this time that Dali fully launched her personal training business quitting her 5-year corporate IT job and began coaching women online and in her community. While writing this book she also recertified as a CPT and became a Certified Weight Management Specialist and Certified Group Fitness Instructor.

Dali enjoys Friday movie nights with the family and traveling. She enjoys learning more about what motivates people to act as well as continually learning about optimal health, weight loss, and how the gut plays a role in our metabolism and hormonal changes.

She enjoys coaching women using an online and hybrid model through her *Defeat It!* mobile app, website, and Facebook.

During her spare time, Dali enjoys singing and volunteering in the Worship Band at her local church on Sundays.

To book Dali for speaking engagements, request personal training and nutrition services, or send your *Defeat IT!* testimonial, visit www.daliburgado.com.

Works Cited

Campbell, Heather J. Leidy and Wayne W. 2011. "The Effect of Eating Frequency on Appetite Control and Food Intake: Brief Synopsis of Controlled Feeding Studies." *The Journal of Nutrition* 157. http://jn.nutrition.org/content/141/1/154.full.pdf+html.

Denjean, Cecile. 2013. *The Gut: Our Second Brain.* Gaia TV. https://www.gaia.com/video/gut-our-second-brain.

Diguilio, Sarah. 2017. "7 Signs You Need To Eat More To Lose Weight." *Prevention Magazine*, May 2. http://www.prevention.com/weight-loss/not-eating-enough-for-weight-loss.

Farmer, Adam D., Holly A. Randall, and Qasim Aziz. 2014. "It's a gut feeling: How the gut microbiota affects the state." *The Journal of Physiology* 2981–2988. https://www.ncbi.nlm.nih.gov/pmc/articles/PMC4214654/pdf/tjp0592-2981.pdf.

Hellwig, Jennifer Pitzi, Linda D. Meyers, and Jennifer J. Otten, eds. "Dietary Reference Intakes Essential Guide Nutrient Requirements." The National Academies of Sciences, Engineering, and Medicine, September 15, 2006. Accessed June 1, 2017. http://nationalacademies.org/hmd/Reports/2006/Dietary-Reference-Intakes-Essential-Guide-Nutrient-Requirements.aspx.

Kim MS, Hwang SS, Park EJ, Bae JW. 2013. "Strict vegetarian diet improves the risk factors associated with metabolic diseases by modulating gut microbiota and reducing intestinal inflammation." *Environmental Microbiology Reports* 765-75. https://www.ncbi.nlm.nih.gov/pubmed/24115628.

2016. "Medical Definition of Metabolism." *MedicineNet.com* Web. http://www.medicinenet.com/script/main/art.asp?articlekey=4359.

2017. *MedicineNet.com.* Jan 25. Accessed June 1, 2017. http://www.medicinenet.com/script/main/art.asp?articlekey=16619.

n.d. *National Fiber Council.* Accessed 2017. http://www.nationalfibercouncil.org/af_are.shtml.

n.d. *National Fiber Council.* Accessed June 2, 2017. http://www.nationalfibercouncil.org/fiber-female-36-50.shtml.

n.d. *NIH, National Institutes of Health.* Accessed June 1, 2017. "The Human Microbiome Project." http://hmpdacc.org/.

Resta, Robert. 2017. "Am I Man Or Am I A Microbe?" *The DNA Exchange Blog*, March 12: 1. https://thednaexchange.com/tag/total-number-of-bacteria-in-the-human-body/.

Sonnenburg, Justin PhD, and Erica PhD Sonnenburg. 2015. *The Good Gut Taking Control of Your Weight, Your Mood, and Your Long-Term Health.* New York: Penguin Books.

Taylor, Julie. 2016. "Bacterium of the Month: Akkermansia muciniphila." *UBiome Blog*, August 26: Web. http://www.ubiomeblog.com/akkermansiamuciniphila/.

Appendix (Meal Plan Including 25 grams of Fiber)

Food	Calories	Fiber (grams)
Breakfast		
Whole-grain cereal (1 cup)	110	4
Low-fat (1%) milk (1 cup)	120	
Banana (1 medium)	105	3
Lunch		
Tuna on whole wheat	390	3.8
Baby carrots (10)	40	3
Pear (medium w. peel)	80	4
Snack		
Strawberry yogurt (6 oz.)	90	
Dinner		
Grilled salmon (4 oz.)	240	
Spinach (1/2 cup)	20	3
Brown rice (1/2 cup)	108	1.8
Chopped tomato (1 med)	22	1
Snack		
Grapes (1 cup)	104	1.4
Low-fat (1%) milk	120	
		25 grams

Adapted from the National Fiber Council Fiber Calculator for a woman under 50 needing 1700 calories (National Fiber Council 2017).

Download all resources at: https://defeatitbook.com/workbook

Notes

_____

_____

_____

_____

_____

_____

_____

_____

_____

_____

_____

_____

_____

_____

_____

_____

_____

_____

_____

_____

_____

_____

_____

_____

_____

Notes

Notes

_____

_____

_____

_____

_____

_____

_____

_____

_____

_____

_____

_____

_____

_____

_____

_____

_____

_____

_____

_____

_____

Notes

_____

_____

_____

_____

_____

_____

_____

_____

_____

_____

_____

_____

_____

_____

_____

_____

_____

_____

_____

_____

_____

_____

_____

_____

Your *Defeat It!* Testimonial

Before reading Dali's *"Defeat It!"* I

_____

_____

_____

_____

_____

Now, after having read *Defeat It!* I feel/believe/see

_____

_____

_____

_____

_____

Dali's *Defeat It!* book has changed how

_____

_____

_____

_____

_____

Thank you for your purchasing *Defeat It!* Please use add your testimonial and review on Amazon or send this to me at daliburgadofitness@daliburgado.com. You can use this as an outline for a video testimony as well.

www.ingramcontent.com/pod-product-compliance
Lightning Source LLC
Chambersburg PA
CBHW060859280326
41934CB00007B/1115